Hungry for More

A Keeping-It-Real Guide for Black Women on Weight and Body Image

Robyn McGee

FOREWORD BY M. JOYCELYN ELDERS, MD

SEAL PRESS

HUNGRY FOR MORE

A Keeping-It-Real Guide for Black Women
on Weight and Body Image

Published by
Seal Press
An Imprint of
Avalon Publishing Group, Incorporated
1400 65th Street, Suite 250
Emeryville, CA 94608

ISBN-10 1-58005-149-9
ISBN-13 978-1-58005-149-1

9 8 7 6 5 4 3 2 1

Library of Congress Cataloging-in-Publication Data
McGee, Robyn.
Hungry for more : a keeping-it-real guide for Black women on weight and body
image / by Robyn McGee.
p. cm.
Includes bibliographical references.
ISBN 1-58005-149-9
1. Obesity in women--Prevention. 2. African American women--Health and
hygiene. 3. Body image in women. 4. Brakefield, Carolyn Cathy, 1951-2001-
-Death. 5. Overweight women--Biography. 6. Gastric bypass--Patients--
Biography. 7. Gastric bypass--Complications. I. Title.
RC628.M374 2005
616.3'98'0082--dc22
2005018661

Cover and interior design by Patrick David Barber
Printed in the United States of America by Worzalla
Distributed by Publishers Group West

Some names have been changed to protecct the privacy of individuals.

Valeria E. Molkew
March 7th, 2007

For Cathy.
Rest in Peace in God's Arms.

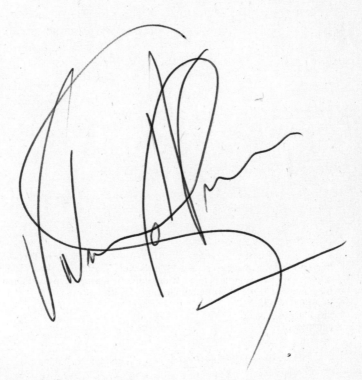

Table of Contents

Foreword

ROBYN MCGEE'S *Hungry for More: A Keeping-It-Real Guide for Black Women on Weight and Body Image* is a groundbreaking examination of African American women and the issue of obesity. In recounting the tragedy of her own sister's lifelong battle with her weight, and her untimely death, Robyn has put forth important ideas about how and why black women struggle with health issues and what can be done so that African Americans and all women can lead longer, more productive lives. Today, thousands of women like Cathy, her sister, are seeking a quick fix in the form of weight-loss surgery and cosmetic surgery. However, what appears to be an easy solution can result in disaster — even death. Oftentimes, a simple change in attitude — heightening self-love and self-acceptance — can prevent the need for life-risking surgeries and lead the way to healthier lifestyles.

Being healthy physically and emotionally go hand in hand. Robyn argues that many black women, like Cathy, suffer from undiagnosed depression, which can lead to binge eating, anorexia, bulimia, and other eating disorders. In addition, child-hood sexual abuse and internalized racism are other factors Robyn explains contribute to the high incidences of overweight and obese black women.

The notion that black women are "satisfied" being over-weight has caused both the society at large and the medical com-munity in particular to ignore the risks of carrying around extra weight. Although being overweight or obese does not automati-cally mean being unhealthy, these conditions can contribute to life-threatening diseases, as Robyn points out.

We must have a comprehensive health education in our schools that includes nutrition education. Improved education is crucial in enabling African Americans to avoid life-threaten-ing diseases, such as obesity, heart disease, hypertension, cancer, stroke, and HIV/AIDS. Not only should health and physical edu-cation be taught from kindergarten through eighth grade in every school in America, but a comprehensive program of information and awareness should be made available to all American families through public service announcements and other public forums.

In addition, public policy plays a necessary role in solving the heath challenges in this country. Promoting preventative health care and making quality heathcare affordable, available, and accessible to working families are steps in the right direction.

Hungry for More gives a new urgency to the much-needed dia-logue in the African American community about the importance of physical education and good nutrition in the battle against weight-related, preventable illnesses. *Hungry for More* also lets black women, schools, policymakers, and our community know that we need help — and that they can help make it happen.

— M. JOYCELYN ELDERS, MD
FORMER U.S. SURGEON GENERAL
AUGUST 2005

Why I Wrote *Hungry for More*

BEFORE DAYBREAK ON April 16, 2001, a few days after Easter, I received a phone call that changed my life. I learned that my beloved older sister, Carolyn "Cathy" Brakefield, was dead. Less than a week before, Cathy had gone to the hospital to fulfill her lifelong dream of losing weight. But something went terribly wrong. She died from complications related to gastric bypass surgery.

Just forty-nine years old, Cathy left a husband and four children, shocked and devastated parents, a large extended family, and lifelong friends. Cathy's efforts to stabilize her marriage and lose weight had become a nightmare, and we were left with a million "whys." Less than a month after she received insurance approval to have the operation, she went under the knife. Why did everything happen so fast? Didn't the doctors know Cathy's heart condition made her a poor candidate for this kind of surgery? What kind of counseling did Cathy receive? Why didn't her husband talk her out of having the operation? Why was Cathy so willing to gamble with her life to lose weight?

"Either I will die on the operating table or die from being

fat," Cathy said before her operation, referring to the high blood
pressure and heart disease she was managing with medication.
Her words chilled me. In Cathy's mind those were her only two
choices.

In 2001, gastric bypass, also known as "bariatric" (meaning weight),
surgery wasn't nearly as popular as it is today. At the time of Cathy's
death, a few high-profile celebrities, like singer Carnie Wilson, were
lauding the surgery. But little was written or reported about the
downside of the operation — its high mortality rate, the incidence
of additional surgeries needed to trim excess fat, the likelihood of
regaining the lost weight over time. Suddenly the media was full
of newly skinny folks claiming to have lost one hundred pounds or
more after the surgery. Their get-thin-quick declarations were simply too seductive for countless Americans who suffer from obesity
(and profit-minded insurance companies and surgeons) to resist.

In 2004, nearly 150,000 people had gastric bypass operations,
a much higher number than ever before. As new, less invasive
surgical techniques are developed, weight-loss operations are
increasingly popular. Among the hundreds of thousands of people
undergoing the procedures are a growing number of black women
and even children (as young as eleven years old).

In the years following Cathy's death, I cringed every time I saw
Carnie Wilson. I railed against what I called "that surgery,"

particularly when speaking to the young women of color I meet in my position as the director of the Women's Resource Center at California State University, Dominguez Hills. Many of these young people constantly worry about their weight.

I tell them how Cathy suffered and died and why her death could have been avoided. I advise them to work on improving their self-esteem and furthering their education. From there, better physical and emotional health is sure to follow. I tell them if something looks too good to be true, it probably is.

I've found from years of talking to young women that the more I shared Cathy's story, the more I was encouraged to write *Hungry for More*. At first I had reservations, concerned that my parents, William and Orelda, who had already suffered so much, would be hurt by having to relive what happened to Cathy. I did not want to do anything to cause them more pain. But I began to see the connections between Cathy's battle with her weight and the broader issue of African American women and obesity. I made up my mind to write *Hungry for More* as a tribute to Cathy's life and death, and a cautionary tale for people grappling with decisions about their weight. My family agreed.

According to a study conducted by the Centers for Disease Control and Prevention (CDC), at the turn of the century, an estimated 30 percent of U.S. adults ages twenty and older — nearly 59 million people — were obese, defined as having a body mass index (BMI) of 30 or more. (See Chapter One for an explanation of how BMI is calculated.) The study found that 64 percent of U.S. adults ages twenty and older were overweight, with a BMI of 25 or more.

The problem of obesity stretches across age, racial, ethnic, geographic, and economic boundaries. People are growing increasingly concerned about the incidence of obesity among our children. According to the 1999–2000 National Health and Nutrition Examination Survey (conducted by the CDC), 10 percent of two- to five-year-olds and 15 percent of six- to nineteen-year-olds in the United States are overweight.

One Los Angeles teacher became so worried about one of her students that she threatened to call Child Protective Services about the 270-pound fourteen-year-old if his mother didn't put him on a diet.

Though obesity is a major health concern for many Americans, *Hungry for More* focuses specifically on African Americans because, as a black woman, I am most familiar with the unique challenges we face trying to stay healthy. According to the CDC, 70 percent of black women are overweight or obese. The high numbers may reflect the fact that black people tend to have larger body frames; some in the medical field suggest the "recommended weight" charts should be altered to account for the African American body type. But even with recalculated weight charts, obesity remains a serious threat to African Americans, who rank first among all women in weight-related diseases like breast cancer, hypertension, heart disease, and stroke.

In contrast to the dire health statistics, black women are making tremendous gains in education and employment. A U.S.

Census Bureau study released in March 2005 made headlines when it reported that black and Asian women with bachelor's degrees earn more than white women with similar educations.

Black Power Inc., written by Cora Daniels, and *Having It All?* by Veronica Chambers, are two excellent books that discuss the new generation of educated black women living large and making their mark in the corporate world. Oprah Winfrey, tennis superstars Venus and Serena Williams, Secretary of State Condoleezza Rice, and Patricia E. Bath, inventor of a revolutionary form of laser cataract surgery and the first African American woman to receive a medical patent, are a few examples of black women who have reached levels of worldwide acclaim unimaginable a few generations ago.

In addition, surveys that measure self-image among young women reveal that African Americans report having the most satisfaction with their body type, even when they are bigger than society's definition of "average." It is truly the best of times and the worst of times for black women.

This conundrum obscures the full impact of obesity and weight-related dangers that many black women face. My goal in *Hungry for More* is to examine how popular culture and social paradigms shape the perceptions of black women, and to offer ways that we can feel good about ourselves while still striving for physical and emotional well-being and maintaining a healthy weight.

Being neither a medical doctor nor a fitness expert, I cannot offer ways to lose weight, beyond the basics — eat less, exercise more, drink lots of water, lower your stress. As a writer who has worked inside the advertising industry, a journalist, and a teacher, I look at women and body image through the prism of consumerism, cultural constructs, marketing, and the pervasive power of media that deluges women of all races with the impossible ideal of "the perfect woman" — size 4! Even though black women have traditionally enjoyed a better self-image than other women, many of us are as vulnerable as anyone else to the tyranny of perfection, as we'll explore in Chapter Three.

Media influence aside, for many black women access to quality, affordable health care in our communities is a serious issue. Despite professional success (and the benefits that go with it) in corporate America for some, nearly 39 percent of families headed by single black women live in poverty, and one million black women with children have no health insurance. Without the ability to prevent and treat weight-related diseases before they become major problems, many black women are already at a tremendous disadvantage. Said one young African American woman, who is getting ready to graduate from college and has no medical benefits, "If I could afford to go to the doctor, I would be beautiful."

I am blessed to work on an urban college campus as an advisor to many intelligent, talented, reach-for-the-stars young women of color. Unfortunately, I also witness the harmful obsession girls of all races have about wanting to "be skinny." I hear Cathy's story from the lips of many outwardly confident girls who hate their bodies and are uncomfortable in their own skin. I hear the pain and shame of overweight and obese women who grow increasingly frustrated with each failed fad diet. Some girls try starving themselves, "fasting" to lose weight. Others become so frustrated, they consume too much sugar and salt, grease and booze. Too many of them seek refuge in diet pills, debit-card shopping, Ecstasy, weed, cigarettes, nightclubs, and the wrong men, rather than honestly exploring the reasons they overeat in the first place.

Reality shows like MTV's *I Want a Famous Face* and *Dr. 90210*, about Beverly Hills plastic surgeons and their patients, don't help. Young women now fantasize about having overnight miracles in the form of liposuction, tummy tucks, breast augmentation or reduction, nose jobs, and weight-loss operations. To them, surgery is the most logical way to correct nature's flaws and overcome bad eating habits. Surgery is a shortcut to winning the fight with fat.

Terri, a health-care worker, experienced a personal crisis in college and spent a semester's worth of financial aid on liposuction. Thousands of dollars awarded to her for books and living expenses to help her get through school instead paid for her makeover in a desperate attempt to win her lover back. Terri's lover did not come back, but the fat did during a very stressful time in her life. It was a move she will always regret.

Both the public and private sectors have grown more and more interested in gastric bypass operations as a way of reversing soaring obesity rates. In 2004, Louisiana's state government began offering no-cost gastric bypasses for government employees.

Dr. Walter Poires, a gastric bypass surgeon at East Carolina

University and past president of the American Society for Bariatric Surgery, has been performing these operations for twenty-five years. He and his staff currently do ten free gastric bypass surgeries each week for poor black women. Dr. Poires believes that while women in urban areas may choose gastric bypass as a way to lose weight for cosmetic reasons, the operations are a matter of life and death for the women he treats.

"In some parts of the United States there are well-to-do young women who may be 150 pounds overweight but are otherwise pretty healthy," he says. "These women will pay money out of their own pockets to have a gastric bypass. But people are poor in this area and we live a different kind of life. With our patients weight is not the problem; the problem is the associated diseases. For example, women come to us with diabetes or heart failure or they're disabled by arthritis; those are the people we operate on."

Within a day of having the ninety-minute operation, a diabetic woman "would no longer have to use insulin," continues Dr. Poires. "Within ten to twelve days that woman would be totally free of diabetes. . . . In some patients, asthma disappears in six days — just goes away. Medicaid pays for these operations because it makes a big difference in people's health."

With those kinds of results, it's hard for me to argue against weight-loss surgery. The premise of *Hungry for More* is not to dismiss gastric bypass as an option. The choice of whether to seek that operation is a personal decision. Instead, I strongly encourage women considering the surgical route to get as much counseling *before and after* they go through with it. My message in *Hungry for More* is this: Unless we change what's in our hearts and minds, no amount of surgery will make us feel whole. Without psychological change to go with our physical change, we could risk gaining all the weight back.

Also critical to surgery's success is adequate professional medical attention. Gastric bypass done on the quick *is* life-threatening. It is essential that we take time, get second opinions, find a doctor we trust. Otherwise we may wind up dying to be thin, like Cathy.

Because so many Americans are fat and looking for answers, hysteria about obesity and the dangers of fast food appear online and on television as frequently as you can type www. While writing *Hungry for More*, I read food-related headlines that ranged from the practical — "Study Ties Dementia, Obesity in Middle Age" and "U.S. Introduces 12 New Food Pyramids" — to the disgusting — "Woman Finds Human Finger in [Fast Food] Chili." At the time of this writing, it appears that the finger-in-the-chili story was a hoax, news that has inspired a collective sigh of relief from the fast food industry.

But the fast food industry is waging a lot of battles these days, particularly when it comes to the issue of obesity. A group of restaurant owners and fast food manufacturers recently set out to counter the federal government's reporting on weight problems. The group asserts that the American public is being misled about the obesity epidemic.

Chafing under criticism and keeping its eye on maintaining profitability and goodwill, fast food and related companies have formed a nonprofit coalition called the Center for Consumer Freedom. In April 2005 the organization launched a ferocious advertising campaign aimed at dismissing as hype the well-publicized concerns about the numbers of Americans dying of obesity.[1]

The group was particularly incensed by a report published in 2004 by the CDC that stated that obesity is "set to take over" smoking in the number of preventable deaths. "Diet and physical inactivity accounted for 400,000 deaths in 2000, or about 16.6 percent of total deaths. Tobacco, with 435,000 deaths, was 18.1 percent of the total."[2]

After the report came out, the CDC admitted that its study was flawed. The National Center for Health Statistics (NCHS), a division of the CDC, put obesity deaths at only a quarter of the number reported in the CDC study. The NCHS attributed the discrepancy to the CDC's reliance on faulty data for its analysis. I agree with the *Los Angeles Times* article that attributed the CDC public relations disaster to "miscommunications, bureaucratic snafus and acquiescence from dissenting scientists."[3]

The mistake attracted a lot of media attention, as well as the attention of the food industry's Center for Consumer Freedom group. In response, it ran full-page ads in *Newsweek* and the *New York Times*, among other publications, skewering the "food police, trial lawyers and our own government," and calling obesity "hype."

While acknowledging the CDC's error about the number of obesity-related deaths, many health-care professionals and educators see this advertising assault by the Center for Consumer Freedom as a way to deliberately muddy the waters and confuse the public.

But some doctors and advocates like the National Association to Advance Fat Acceptance (NAAFA) believe that being overweight or obese does not *automatically* mean a person is in ill health. In fact behavioral scientist Dr. Martin Binks of the Duke Diet & Fitness Center maintains that obese patients are at *greater* risk undergoing weight-loss surgery if they also suffer from comorbidities like hypertension and diabetes. Binks believes that in those cases, ironically, the excess weight may be a safer option than surgery.

It is not the numbers on the scale that hurt us. The harm comes when carrying excess weight increases your risk for diabetes, hypertension, certain cancers, high cholesterol, and other life-threatening illnesses that disproportionately affect black and Latino communities.

My question to the food industry's Center for Consumer Freedom, financing the "Obesity Hype" campaign, is this: Do we believe you, or our own lying eyes?

Hungry for More takes a holistic approach to weight and its health, social, and cultural implications. Threaded throughout is Cathy's story, a personal tragedy, a preventable loss. In Chapter One, "Cathy's Slim Hopes," I introduce my sister and describe the battle with her weight that ended her life.

Chapter Two, "From the Motherland to Mickey D's," explores the history of obesity in the African American community. Chapter Three, "Can a Big Sister Get Some Love?" examines plus-size women and their relationships, both romantic and familial. Chapter Four, "Digging Our Graves with Our Forks," takes a look at some of the most common reasons for overeating: a way of coping with the pain of abuse, a manifestation of depression, an addiction to food.

Chapter Five, "Big Girls in La-La Land," surveys how big black women are portrayed in popular culture through movies, song, and literature, from Aunt Jemima to the positive personas of large and lovely stars such as Queen Latifah and Mo'Nique.

Chapter Six, "Keeping Secrets, Taking Risks," examines the nuts and bolts of gastric bypass, its potential risks, and the aftermath many patients face, which seems to get obscured in the excitement of what is a remedy at best, a quick fix at worst. Dr. Mal Fobi, the inventor of the popular Fobi pouch method of weight-loss surgery — nicknamed "Surgeon to the Stars" because of his celebrity patients, including comedian Roseanne, jazz great Etta James, and *American Idol*'s Randy Jackson — shares insights about how even now, twenty years after beginning to acknowledge obesity as a health problem, the medical profession still knows very little about how to treat and prevent obesity.

Chapter Seven, "Latinas: Our Bodies, Ourselves," compares the challenges African American women share with Latinas, in terms of body image and social pressures, and offers ways to break through to better education and healthier lifestyle choices.

In Chapter Eight, "Before You Make the Call," I offer suggestions for taking a different path to healthy weight. I avoid telling women to diet in *Hungry for More* for the simple reason that diets per se do not work.

And finally, "Generation XXXL," the last chapter, focuses on black children who are big and getting bigger, and ways to stop this epidemic now. We need to give our kids the opportunity to live lives that are longer and healthier than our own.

Years ago when I was vacationing in Montego Bay, a young Jamaican brother asked me a question for the ages: "Why do black women get mad when you call them fat?" He was truly mystified. I explained that, for many of us, being called fat is an insult, even if it is true.

That said, I occasionally use the word "fat," not as a diss but as a description. Women who describe themselves as fat say if I really want to keep it real and break through the denial, I should call it the way it is. And, although it may be politically correct, it would also be disingenuous to dance around a word the whole world uses.

Nor can I dance around the fact that Cathy didn't need to die. Her life lessons are at the core of *Hungry for More*. I am honored to share with the world her bittersweet gifts to me. If reading *Hungry for More* causes even one woman who struggles with her weight to pass a mirror and not lower her head, but smile, my mission is accomplished.

— ROBYN "ROB" McGEE
JUNE 2005

CHAPTER ONE

Cathy's Slim Hopes

Now at last, Cathy is thin.

—FROM THE EULOGY FOR CAROLYN "CATHY" BRAKEFIELD,
September 28, 1951–April 16, 2001

MY SISTER CATHY loved a good party.

The last time I saw Cathy she was hosting a friend's wedding. Champagne glass in hand, her head thrown back laughing, she was raising the roof with longtime and newly found friends. Food enough for ten armies — pounds of baked ham, platters of macaroni and cheese, buttered rolls, plus endless wine — all Cathy's favorite dishes were on the menu that night.

Younger by four years, I grew up in awe of Cathy. I am Nikes and braids and have been accused by other family members of "squeezing a dollar until the eagle hollers." Cathy, on the other hand, was pink manicures and diamonds big enough for a drama queen, her hair always perfectly coiffed and woven with

1

rich brunette highlights. Money burned a hole in her designer bags. Cathy worked hard as an in-home childcare provider. And she played hard too: drop-of-the-hat trips up the California coast to watch the sunset with her husband of fifteen years; all-day shopping with her two oldest daughters; and gathering as many loved ones as would fit in a rented limo to ride to the Hyatt for Sunday brunch.

Folks always ask me about her size. How big was Cathy? I suppose they expect me to describe a two-ton oddity like someone you might see on the *Jerry Springer Show*. Cathy was light-years away from that. To me, she was built the way many black women are: wide hips, thick legs and thighs, and a full tummy and bosom. At first glance, she looked closer to fifty pounds over-weight than the one hundred extra pounds she carried — weight that eventually qualified her for gastric bypass surgery. She was fly and fashionable on the outside, but inside she was tormented by her weight and hungry for relief.

A few weeks before her friend's wedding celebration, my youngest sister, Theresa, and I sat with Cathy in a restaurant toasting Cathy's future. I think back on that afternoon as "Cathy's last luncheon." Her plate of hot wings remained untouched as she spoke excitedly about how she was going to be "a size 9 by the big 5-0," referring to her upcoming fiftieth birthday and waving her arms with a diva's flair. Her plan was to shrink from size 26 to a third that size. Cathy swore she had finally found a way to lose one hundred pounds — and to keep it off forever.

Breaking bread with my sisters that afternoon, I thought back to a time when we were children gathered for Sunday dinner with my three other sisters, Pat, Claudia, and Sheilah, my brother William, Mom, and Dad. Our childhood diet included a hefty combination of delicacies from Mom's homeland of Panama: fried dough called *bakes*, Spanish-flavored *arroz con pollo*, oil-cooked plantains, salty sea bass cooked in tomato sauce, peas, and rice. We also munched Southern-style fried chicken, mashed potatoes with gravy, ham hocks, cornbread, and hot buttered rolls — foods reflecting Dad's Mississippi heritage. Growing up in a home with both Latino and African American influences meant we relished delicious, fattening foods from two distinct cultures.

My sisters and I get our thick body types from my dad. Mom, on the other hand, had the exact opposite problem. Born in the Central American country of Costa Rica and raised in neighboring Panama, Mom was so thin, her elder relatives used to say, "A strong wind might swoop her up and blow her away." Mom is still petite into her seventies, while the rest of us are what African Americans lovingly call "healthy."

Watching Cathy that day in the restaurant, I remember thinking, "How are you going to be a size 9? You've never been a size 9." I did not voice my concerns aloud.

Cathy beamed, describing singer Carnie Wilson's *People* magazine cover story about her operation that reduced the size of her stomach. Cathy told us it was called "gastric bypass weight-loss surgery," and that "with the right medical insurance, anyone could have one, not just celebrities." It sounded risky, but I knew it was pointless to try to talk her out of it. Cathy's mind was set; her eyes sparkled like the bling on her fingers. Victory was near.

After a lifetime of battling her weight, Cathy was finally going to be skinny.

"With my operation, I'll be able to only eat cupfuls of food. I'll never be fat again," Cathy told us proudly. We shrugged and accepted her latest thin hope, few questions asked. I had no idea what she was getting into. I figured the operation would be no more dangerous than an appendectomy or a tummy tuck. Easy, simple, routine.

A few weeks after our afternoon together, my beloved sister was dead. Cathy was just forty-nine years old.

The coroner listed the cause of death as "cardiac arrest" on Cathy's autopsy. I found out later (thanks to the medical records our attorney subpoenaed for our lawsuit) that Cathy developed a post-surgery infection, common in gastric bypass patients. The contamination taxed Cathy's heart, already weakened by hardening of the arteries, beginning diabetes, and hypertension. Funny the things you learn from an autopsy, the ultimate physical. None of us had any idea Cathy was a borderline diabetic.

Cathy suffered for four days and never made it out of Temple Hospital. The struggle with her weight was finally over, visions of a new life laid to rest.

Surgery Numbers Swell

Gastric bypass surgeries have increased dramatically in recent years, jumping more than 500 percent worldwide in the last eleven years, from 16,800 operations in 1993 to 140,640 in 2004, according to the American Society for Bariatric Surgery. African Americans make up 9 percent of those patients, and the average age is around thirty-nine, according to data compiled by the International Bariatric Registry. (Most gastric bypass patients across all ethnicities are women, but the number of men seeking this procedure is starting to catch up.)

Plastic surgery used to be frowned on in the African American community. "Being cut" tapped into both a mistrust of the medical profession (see Chapter Six) and an aversion to altering one's features to look "more white" (Michael Jackson predictably comes up in that discussion). But high-profile celebrities, like singing legend Patti LaBelle, have made so-called surgical makeovers more acceptable among blacks. In just two years, the number of black cosmetic surgery patients has grown by almost one-third, according to the American Society of Plastic Surgeons, jumping from 375,025 in 2002 to 487,887 in 2004.

Driven by what I call the three m's — movies, magazines, and mania for the "perfect look" — many blacks are opting for nose jobs, cheek implants, eye surgery to remove lines and bags, butt lifts, breast enlargements, and tummy tucks.

Gastric bypass surgery is far more serious than a cut and fold, however. Desperate to be thin, women like Cathy are willing to risk their lives having their stomachs cut and reconfigured. These women see surgery as a shortcut to ridding themselves of all their problems along with pounds of fat. Many, like Cathy, are sick and tired of feeling bad and believe that life before weight-loss surgery is a mere dress rehearsal and that real life begins once they are thin. Like Cathy, they are frustrated with pills and powders, Weight Watchers meetings, Fen-Phen warnings, grapefruit diets, Atkins attempts, NutriSystem, OPTIFAST, or traveling to places like Tijuana or Canada to buy miracle injections of appetite suppressants. They view weight-loss surgery as a magic bullet, a symbol for taking control of their lives, a renewal of hope. They consider hair loss, additional surgeries, and eating complications after gastric bypass operations a small price to pay to be thin.

Fortunately, most people who undergo gastric bypass will not die. Weight-loss surgeons quote the mortality rate as one death out of every two hundred patients. But a study by the University of Washington cites an even scarier statistic: one death in every fifty, when taking into account all weight-loss surgery patients at all hospitals that will suffer and die from various surgery-related complications such as blood clots, fluid leakage, and infections. In addition, the people who want the surgery most — those with so-called "comorbidities," such as diabetes and heart disease — face the greatest risk of having something go wrong.[1]

Wake-Up Call

In late 2000, a few months before Cathy died, *EBONY* magazine, the most reliable mirror of African American culture, ran a story about black women and obesity that delivered a wake-up call about the burgeoning crisis. According to the article, 70 percent of the more than 18 million black women in America are considered obese or overweight.

Doctors use a formula known as the "body mass index" (BMI) — calculated by using an equation that divides weight by height — to determine a person's ideal weight. BMI correlates with body fat. For example, you are considered "overweight" if your BMI measures 25 or above. Consequently, a woman who is five foot four and weighs 145 pounds is considered overweight. "Obesity" is defined as a BMI of 30 or above — for instance, someone who is five foot four and 175 pounds.

But BMI isn't such a reliable gauge for blacks. We tend to have bigger body frames and bigger bones than the average white person, according to Dr. Mal Fobi, inventor of the popular Fobi pouch method of weight-loss surgery. "Therefore blacks can weigh more, relatively speaking," Dr. Fobi suggests. He states that the height/weight charts most doctors rely on should differentiate between black and white women. If calibrated specifically to blacks, the "norm for African American women would mean an added twenty-five or thirty pounds to the current BMI designations."

The current BMI weight standards label more black women overweight, qualifying them for the weight threshold they must meet to be eligible for weight-loss surgery. (Some women have figured out creative ways to get around this threshold, as will be discussed in Chapter Six.

Recently there has been more talk of reconfiguring the BMI to account for differing musculature and other factors. It follows the revelation that by the current BMI standard, many rock-solid athletes, including basketball superstar Shaquille O'Neal, are considered overweight.

Even with a redefined BMI that more accurately reflects the black physique, obesity is still a major threat to many African Americans' health. Cathy's autopsy listed her as being "morbidly obese," meaning she had a BMI of 40 or above. According to doctors, "morbid" is a medical term that refers to obesity-related diseases like diabetes or hypertension that increase dramatically when a particular weight is reached.[2]

Recent studies by the American Obesity Association reveal that heart disease and stroke, diabetes, osteoporosis, hypertension, cancer, and other weight-related illnesses send black women to their graves years earlier than other women. We lead all women in weight-related illnesses, with nearly three out of four black women considered overweight or obese.

When the California Black Women's Health Project conducted a study in 2001 to determine the state of black women's physical and emotional health, they asked black women to prioritize their health concerns. With the exception of the seventeen- to nineteen-year-olds, women reported weight as their primary worry. In light of these and similar studies, health-care professionals — including physicians, mental health professionals, educators, nutritionists, and physical fitness experts — have mobilized to reverse the deadly trend of poor health among African Americans. Black churches, community groups, hospitals, colleges, and universities around the country now regularly host wellness forums, events devoted to education about and prevention of maladies that disproportionately affect the black community, such as cigarette smoking, hypertension, prostate, colon, and breast cancer, diabetes, HIV/AIDS, and obesity.

In 2005, TV host and best-selling author Tavis Smiley presented a panel discussion on the state of the health of black Americans, which was broadcast around the world on C-SPAN. Featured on that program were prominent black women associated with wellness, including former U.S. Surgeon General Dr. Joycelyn Elders, fitness expert Donna Richardson Joyner, and Olympic champion Jackie Joyner-Kersee. All three women were unequivocal about what it will take for African Americans to live healthier lives: education, education, and more education.

Awareness and action are critical if we are to improve our health and increase the quality *and* quantity of life for black people. Currently, life expectancy for black women is 75.5 years versus 80.2 years for white females. The statistics are even grimmer for black males, whose life expectancy is 68.6 years versus 75.0 years for white men.

African Americans are worldwide leaders in politics, religion, business, entertainment, and sports. Maintaining the momentum from the civil rights struggles of the 1950s and '60s and the fight for economic empowerment of the '80s and '90s, the twenty-first century should be the time when we as a community make the commitment to living longer, healthier lives by reducing obesity and weight-related illnesses.

Unless current trends are reversed, many black women now breaking down racial and gender barriers in the workplace may find that ill health during their prime dashes their chance to fulfill their dreams. A proactive stance will ensure that our children, also the most obese group among young people (see Chapter Nine, "Generation XXXL"), do not suffer from preventable diseases and premature deaths.

What's Eating Her?

Hungry for More is about the physical and social aspects of weight as perceived by those inside and outside the black community in light of our current health crisis. As we black women take responsibility for improved fitness and maintaining a healthy weight, we recognize that being overweight is about more than overeating. As an advisor to college-aged women for the past eight years, I've noticed a shift in the ideal of beauty among both young men and young women of color. Image-makers and marketers pummel the public with the relentless stereotype of the perfect woman as thin and hyperenergetic, with pearly white teeth, flawless skin, and long hair.

In the past, African Americans have rejected the skin-and-bones, anorexic, adolescent boy–shaped standard of beauty popular with white women since the Victorian era. "Big Mama" was the persona we in the black community idolized. A full-figured grandmother whose body reflected the abundance of her wisdom, Big Mama served as a symbol of a lifetime of strength and sacrifice for the entire race.

Today, the media-created "video ho" — flighty, hypersexual, fat-free vixen — has replaced Big Mama as the commercial representation of black womanhood. As more and more young women are indoctrinated and surrounded by the video ho as icon, they compare themselves to what they see on cable TV, on the silver screen, and in popular youth-oriented publications like *XXL* and *VIBE*. Girls and young women, not yet comfortable with themselves, feel pressured to measure up to an impossible paradigm. As a result, many develop destructive behaviors, including eating disorders (e.g., compulsive overeating, anorexia, and bulimia), and increasingly choose surgical solutions.

Because my background is in journalism and black studies, I approach black women's health issues from the perspective of the historical and popular cultural forces that shape who we are. Having watched my sister Cathy and other women struggle with weight and self-image, I realize the challenge of being healthy and satisfied with the way we look — both the way we see ourselves and the way others see us — can last a lifetime.

Black women struggle with a dichotomy that I believe has until recently obscured the weight-related issues that negatively affect our health. For example, in a 2001 study of women and self-image conducted at Northwestern University, the researchers found that white women with a BMI of 25 or more expressed dissatisfaction with their bodies. Black women, by contrast, didn't express dissatisfaction with their bodies until they approached a BMI of 30, the threshold for obesity.[3] Studies like these do not tell the whole story. Deluged with celluloid images of lithe women being so desirable, more and more black women are rejecting the large and lovely Big Mama persona. While we still express positivity about our bodies, we believe the grass is greener on the skinny side, and increasingly black women are hoping to cross over.

Happily over the past ten years our weight problems have been taken more seriously. It's a wonderful thing that as African Americans we take pride in being "big, beautiful women." However, it is important to understand that carrying extra weight can cause life-threatening harm.

Black women and others have weight problems for a variety of reasons. Genetics, poverty, food addictions, depression, psychological traumas, such as sexual abuse, and lack of exercise contribute to the "epidemic" of obesity in the United States, now considered the "fattest place on earth."

Unique to African Americans are additional factors: our physiological makeup, the historical relationship between African Americans and eating (including the "soul food" diet), the absence of exercise in our daily lives, and the black community's mistrust of and lack of access to the medical profession.

Being fat is neither a moral failing nor a life sentence. The idea that people need only to "push away from the table and put their fork down" is ignorant and short-sighted. The choice is not between doing nothing and having radical stomach surgery. Instead we can reach for the happy medium between self-acceptance and working toward self-improvement.

Magic Wands and Reality Checks

Popular television host Montel Williams wrote a book called *Mountain, Get Out of My Way*. This title reminds me of the resilience of black women. Being overweight and obese are not problems that occurred overnight, and they will not be solved in a day's time.

In some families, women generation after generation have carried extra weight, leading some to believe that because they may have a so-called "fat gene," they are destined to be overweight no matter what.

The problem of reducing obesity may seem overwhelming. It will take education and dedication to help us to become more physically fit and maintain a healthier weight. Lifestyle changes —including eating our favorite foods in moderation, keeping our stress levels low, and exercising regularly—are stepping stones to optimum health in mind, body, and spirit.

Achieving better health means taking personal responsibility for ourselves and our children to maintain a healthy weight and physical fitness. Public policy also plays an important role for millions of Americans who are overweight and obese. If I had a magic wand I could wave to ding politicians and their corporate allies, I would demand the following:

1. *Offer affordable health insurance to all Americans.* African Americans are the largest group of the medically uninsured in this country. Many of us simply cannot afford to go to the doctor on a regular basis. With preventive health care,

obesity and weight-related diseases like diabetes and hypertension could be diagnosed and treated before they become full blown.

2. *Provide access to quality health-care facilities.* Instead of constructing another Wienerschnitzel or Church's Fried Chicken, which will net multibillion-dollar corporations millions more, encourage corporations to use some of their resources to build wellness clinics that provide ongoing health care and education, and community recreation centers for adults and children. And while they're at it, why not design a few neighborhood centers for group, family, and individual psychological counseling. Being good corporate citizens is easy. A corporate logo will look just as good on a place of healing as it does on a fast food joint.

3. *Restore physical education programs in elementary, middle, and high schools.* According to a *Detroit Daily News* October 2003 article entitled, "More U.S. Schools Cut Gym," four in ten high school students took daily physical education classes fourteen years ago. Today barely a third of students take PE. In 1980, just 5 percent of school-age children were severely overweight; twenty years later, the number had jumped to 15 percent.[4] The correlation between lack of daily physical activity and the rate of obesity among our kids seems obvious. Many physical education classes have been cut to give students more time to study for the Bush administration's education initiatives. Without daily physical education "no child left behind" has become "lots of children with plenty of behind."

4. *Make nutrition education mandatory in K–12.* It is not enough today for kids to see the U.S. Department of Agriculture's flashy new food pyramid (www.mypyramid.gov). They must be educated about how foods affect their bodies. We must *teach* our kids when, what, and how to eat. Nutrition education and PE programs in our schools could substantially reduce obesity for future generations.

Rob's Recommendations

The Black Women's Health Book: Speaking for Ourselves, edited by Evelyn C. White, published by Seal Press, 1994.

Blessed Health: The African-American Woman's Guide to Physical and Spiritual Well-Being, by Melody T. McCloud and Angela Ebron, published by Fireside, 2003.

Dr. Ro's Ten Secrets to Livin' Healthy: America's Most Renowned African American Nutritionist Shows You How to Look Great, Feel Better, and Live Longer by Eating Right, by Rovenia M. Brock, published by Bantam Doubleday Dell, 2003.

Dr. Gavin's Health Guide for African Americans: How to Keep Yourself and Your Children Well, by James R. Gavin, published by the American Diabetes Association, 2004.

Hollywood's Finest

Beauty Shop. Queen Latifah stars as a large and lovely entrepreneur and single mom who wins the heart of Djimon Hounsou. 2005.

The Parkers. Positively hilarious TV sitcom about plus-size single mother Mo'Nique and college-aged daughter Countess Vaughn. 1999–2004.

CHAPTER TWO

From the Motherland to Mickey D's

*As you live, believe in life! Always human beings will live
and progress to greater, broader and fuller life.*
— W.E.B. DUBOIS

WHEN TALKING ABOUT weight issues, women say to me, "Big
Mama lived into her eighties, and she was fat." That may be true,
but things in 2005 are radically different from when our grand-
mothers and great-aunties were coming up. Fat today is more
dangerous than fat was yesterday — our stress levels are higher,
and the food we eat is packaged and processed with more sodium
and other fillers that hurt us more than the food they ate back in
Big Mama's day.

Black people used to eat from the bottom of the food pyramid — more grains, breads, and proteins — because we could
not afford meat for the entire family and would supplement the
little meat we had with lots of beans and rice. Today, however,

overeating and buying junk food have become status symbols. Instead of spending our food budget on balanced meals, we spend it on Kentucky Fried and Pizza Hut.

Physical labor was also a big part of black life before the technological revolution. We worked on farms and in factories; we walked miles and rode bikes; we chopped wood and cleaned houses (our own and other people's); we drew water from the well; we hoed, raked, pushed lawnmowers; we planted gardens and hung clothes in the hot sun. It's important to realize that the current obesity crisis in the black community has long and deep roots. In fact the problem with obesity and African Americans can be traced back to the motherland.

"Black people who are overweight come from deprived great, great ancestors," says Dr. Fobi. "Those people's bodies were trained to survive during times of famine and starvation. Those who were the most deprived developed better abilities to store fat." According to Dr. Fobi, the African race is like other races where people were disadvantaged for a long time so "now that they have too much food, they will store the extra as fat."

Dr. Walter Poires, past president of the American Society of Bariatric Surgery, has conducted numerous studies related to obesity and African Americans and agrees with Dr. Fobi that fat storage differs among races: "The Caucasian woman, when she has an excess of energy as fat, compares more to having a checking account at the bank. That is, when she has to 'draw on it,' it comes out pretty easily. When black women, on the other hand, have an excess of fat, and they store it, [it's] as though the black women put fat into a 'trust fund' meaning it's much more difficult for [them] to get the fat back out."

For some starving populations of black people living in modern-day African societies, the ability to store fat is a plus. However, for the middle-class African American woman eating too much food, the ability to store fat is not an advantage. It is a burden.

The Chitlin Circuit

Even though Queen Califia in Baja California represents the early history of black women on these shores (see "Califia Dreamin'" later in this chapter), many blacks trace their ancestry to Africa. Before slavery, African people enjoyed a relationship with food that included a "god consciousness." According to health educator Anita Roberts at California State University, Dominguez Hills, our African ancestors regarded food in much the same way many vegetarians do today: They believed that all living things including animals have souls and that for a human to ingest an animal borders on the sacrilegious. "Early Africans chose to eat vegetables instead of living creatures, believing foods like yams, for example, held sacred properties, greater than the actual nutrients within," says Roberts. "The 'transfer' of Africans from their homeland to America during the slave trade and along the Middle Passage was when black people lost the component of spirituality with regards to food. We were forced to eat whatever we could just to survive."

The paradoxically nicknamed "soul food" became the primary diet for Africans in America. "Sundays were considered 'days of rest' and the only time enslaved families could gather together to eat with others who were like them," Roberts says. "We ate big meals made from recycled scraps that were thrown away by the white masters. Pig's feet, cow toes, cow brains, and pig intestine 'chitlins' were leftovers from the animals that folks in the 'big house' had killed for food." Being the creative people we are, our forefathers and mothers salvaged these discarded animal parts and created a whole cuisine out of garbage.

Although soul food originated as a matter of survival, black Americans are still paying for the custom today. As tasty and filling as soul food is, it is also rich in fat and salt and is a poor source of nutrition that has been passed from generation to generation.

Fast Food to the Rescue?

In the 1950s, McDonald's Golden Arches beckoned to a new generation of Americans. Soon chain restaurants, imitating McDonald's formula, spread across the land serving fast, high-fat foods at convenient drive-thru windows that let you buy ready-to-eat meals without even needing to park your car and walk inside to get your order. When they first appeared on the American cultural landscape, the major fast food companies — McDonald's, Jack-in-the-Box, Carl's Jr., Taco Bell, and Burger King — avoided opening franchises in black neighborhoods, perhaps fearing they'd be run out by theft and vandalism, but obviously not recognizing the economic force of African Americans. Family barbeque shacks and fried chicken joints already in the community were able to capitalize on black folks' increased appetite for good tasting, cheap, wax-papered, quick, high-calorie meals.

In the 1960s, McDonald's, yielding to pressure from civil rights groups, began selling franchises to black businessmen, and fast food restaurants started to blossom in the inner cities.[1] We even affectionately call McDonald's "Mickey D's," as though he were a lifelong friend. But the arrival of Mickey D's and his buddies, Jack-in-the-Box and Burger King, in minority communities has been a double-edged sword. On one hand, these chains offer employment opportunities and a tax base for poorer neighborhoods.

However, their inexpensive, convenient food is mostly devoid of nutritional value and contributes to the devastating problem of obesity and weight-related diseases among black adults and children alike. Nonetheless, fast food restaurants with bargain-priced menus for the family, ready within minutes, are simply too tempting to pass up. Convenience has a price. Spending twenty bucks or more on fast food every day adds up in terms of dollars, fat, and poor nutrition.

Stress on the Menu

There is no denying that stress levels and harsh economic realities negatively affect the health of black women. Some of us live in neighborhoods where we stay locked indoors praying that stray bullets miss our home and that our loved ones return safely once they leave the house. Walking around the block for exercise is out of the question.

Juggling family matters — not just a spouse and kids, but oftentimes grandchildren or other relatives, as well as aging parents — means that lots of black women have too much on their plates.

Not only did Cathy raise her husband's two daughters, Beth and Katie, from his previous marriage, she and Luke were in the process of adopting two other children at the time she died. Cathy was making great progress with Christopher, a learning-disabled four-year-old who had been in the foster care system. Cathy's youngest adopted daughter, Bekka, was "given" to her by a woman Cathy befriended who was already the single parent of two other kids.

Cathy worked at home, so her house was both her personal and professional space. Her door was literally always open; her three-bedroom house burst at the seams with kids, their parents, assorted guests seeking out Cathy's kind ear or in need of a baby-sitter for their children. Cathy handled her child-rearing duties with joy. But toward the end of her life, all the responsibility began to take its toll, and she took in fewer and fewer kids.

According to the U.S. Census, nearly half of all African American women with children are heads of households. They are more likely to work outside the home and be unable to take time off for sickness or doctor's checkups than their white counterparts. That's if they're lucky enough to be able to afford to go to the doctor. One million black single moms have no health insurance at all. Keeping a roof over our heads and staying healthy is not easy, as we fight off bill collectors while looking for opportunities to better our lives.

In the workplace, black women feel extra pressure to go above and beyond the call of duty, particularly if they are the only minority or female in the higher echelons of a Fortune 500 corporation. With nerves on edge and constant performance demands, many women feel that good eating habits and regular exercise are luxuries they can't afford.

Diane, an African American Hollywood movie producer who has battled a weight problem her entire life, knows that being one minute late for a meeting can blow a deal. With several film scripts in development at one time, Diane works long hours and usually ends up skipping breakfast, "grabbing something quick like burgers and fries for lunch," and devouring it at her desk or while fighting traffic on an L.A. freeway en route to her next appointment.

Once Diane gets home — sometimes as late as midnight — she eats again, right before hitting the sack and without a chance to work off the calories. She sleeps for a few hours and starts the whole hectic routine early the next morning.

High-powered Hollywood executives are not the only black women with poor eating habits. Struggling college students, sisters who are dependent on public assistance for their family needs, and wives and mothers who work either inside or outside of the home all say it is difficult to find the time to exercise and eat a healthy diet. In addition, a significant number of black women live on the edge—homeless, unemployed, drug and alcohol addicted, and fighting with police and the courts for themselves or their children.

Tina is currently "bouncing between my cousin's house and some friends' houses" while looking for a job. "I can't get rid of my 'honey pot,'" Tina says, pointing to the extra fat around her abdomen. "I am homeless but I am gaining weight because I can't eat regular meals and I end up eating junk."

Too often, as black women, we find ourselves physically exhausted, stressed, eating carelessly, and in the words of rapper Tupac Shakur, "hoping it all doesn't fall apart this week." The combination of living a high-anxiety life, eating a steady diet of low-nutrition, high-calorie foods, and not exercising is a recipe for disaster. These are problems not only for black women but for a majority of Americans. Our fat-filled, nervous-wreck, remote-controlled lives will take us out before our time—unless we make necessary changes now.

Since the problem of obesity has become a national crisis, a slew of books and articles has been published, many by well-meaning white academics and journalists who touch on the experience of people of color. Some are better than others. *Fast Food Nation,* written by Eric Schlosser, brilliantly traces the fast food industry's impact not only on American culture but on the worldwide economy as well. Other works, however, use what I call "African Americans as props" stories. For example, *The Obesity*

Myth, by Paul Campos, and the controversial 2000 *Harper's* article "Let Them Eat Fat," by Greg Critser, at first glance seem
empathetic toward African Americans and Latinos regarding the
obesity issue. But beneath the surface, their rhetoric reveals an
attitude toward people of color I find particularly disturbing.

Campos wants us to believe that obesity is really just a cruel
joke concocted by corporate goons to make money. He scoffs at
the notion that "culturally sensitive Public Health intervention
programs to help reduce the high rates of obesity in the black
community encourage black youth to achieve a healthy body
size."[2] Campos also says there is no evidence that connects body
mass and mortality rates in black women.

Even more galling, Critser's article refers to black women as a
"sub-population" and essentially says that rich folk need us to be
fat so they can feel good about themselves.

Wendy Shanker's *A Fat Girl's Guide to Life* (published in 2004)
is even more disappointing. In this self-hating bestseller, Shanker,
a writer for *Us Weekly*, reports that she "wishes she had a dime for
every black man that hit on her," and wonders if their interest in
plus-size women indicates that they'll settle for "sloppy seconds."[3]

I am sure Ms. Shanker did not mean to insult full-figured black
women and Latinas and the men who love them by basically calling
the whole lot of us losers. Shanker uses her positive experiences with
men of color as a way to make a point about acceptance. However,
she ignores the issues African American women and Latinas face
with the triple bigotry we endure being fat, female, and of color.

The conclusions drawn by Shanker, Campos, and Critser

reflect the same straw arguments advanced by the food indus-try's Center for Consumer Freedom — it's not your poundage but your propensity for disease that causes the problem. This further underscores the importance of the black community's search for solutions to our health problems.

A Poor Diet

Economics and health are closely related. According to the American Obesity Association, "Overweight affects African American women and men across all socioeconomic levels. Minority women with low incomes appear to have the great-est likelihood of being overweight. Among Mexican American women, age 20 to 74, the rate of overweight is about 13 percent higher for women living below the poverty line versus above the poverty line."[4]

Supermarket chains that serve affordable nutritious fruits, vegetables, and lean meats are missing from low-income neigh-borhoods. In their place are liquor stores, selling chips, cigarettes, and Chivas Regal. Trying to make food stretch, families cook meals high in fat and starch. Because they feel deprived in other areas, they might reward themselves with cookies, cakes, and other satisfying sweets.

In April 2005, the University of California Cooperative took a positive step toward educating poor families and others about how to deal with obesity. By dialing a toll-free hotline number

(800-514-4494), callers can get answers in English or Spanish to questions such as "Is gastric bypass surgery the answer?" and "Why are the poor more likely to be overweight?"

The friendly recorded voices tell us that research has shown "overweight has replaced malnutrition as the most prevalent nutritional problem among the poor," and "high fat, high sugar foods are the cheapest source of calories for low-income families to buy." For example, french fries at most fast food restaurants cost around a dollar, whereas a single tomato with more nutritional value costs around the same thing.

Crystal and Curves

In a working-class African American neighborhood in Carson, California, twenty-six-year-old Crystal breaks into a cheerleader's smile pointing to her own "before" and "after" snapshots. One captures Crystal as a size 22, the other as a size 4. The manager of a Curves exercise franchise owned by her sister, Crystal spent two years slimming down using the Curves program. Today she is coach, counselor, and conscience to black women trying to reach their physical fitness goals.

Dead-set against all weight-loss surgery, Crystal finally got serious about shedding the excess pounds when her doctor told her she had weak kidneys and wouldn't live to see her children grow up if she didn't adopt a fitness program. That's when Crystal discovered Curves, and her new mission in life.

Many African Americans and Latinas are attracted to Curves' thirty-minutes-a-day, three-times-a-week circuit training in a females-only environment. At the Carson workout facility, Crystal is an exercise evangelical, preaching the value of good nutrition and regular exercise to clients of all ages. She especially targets black women when handing out promotional flyers in the community because even though many sisters are obese, she says, "Black women don't think they need to exercise. They'll say things like, 'My man likes me this way.'"

Crystal understands the emotional pressures many black women face from relationships, jobs, families, and the outside world. So she shares her own success story with her customers and insists that they stick with their three-times-a-week workout for a minimum of six months if they want to see results.

"Two years ago, I could not jog," Crystal says. "So I started walking instead. I went from walking to speed-walking. Now I am able to run five miles three times a week." Crystal tells her clients they must "crawl before they can walk," and they should not expect to be skinny overnight. "It took 'a minute' to put the weight on and it is going to take 'a minute' to take it off," Crystal says. She also gave up sweets and white flour, including breads and pastas.

Crystal observes that many black women who come to Curves blame their weight gain on "blues eating" — snacking because they are bored or stressed, and choosing high-sodium foods, like hot sauce, sweets, and potato chips to satisfy cravings.

Crystal tells her clients that if they must give in to that bag of Doritos or a piece of chocolate cake, or another snack, go ahead and do it. "But if you blow your diet one day, get right back on it the next day," she says. "Women feel that if they cheat on their weight-loss regimen one day, they might as well just give up altogether. But that's not true. You can get right back on the wagon. It's hard to change a lifetime of bad eating habits all at once."

Tom, the husband of an overweight woman who goes through an "I am on a diet" routine about three times a year, complains, "When my wife goes on a diet and stops buying fast food, the whole family has to go on a diet, whether we want to or not. We can't afford to buy different food for everybody, so all of us have to eat her bland and tasteless low-fat food."

Some women use these gripes as excuses to give up their weight-loss plan and revert to the same bad eating habits. Others teach by example; they buy healthy food, show their families how to prepare it, explain to them why they are making these choices, and encourage their loved ones to join in so that the whole family can enjoy better health.

According to Crystal, if you can sacrifice sugary and high-fat snacks and work out at least three times a week, you are on your way to achieving and maintaining an ideal weight. "But for a lot of women, starting an exercise routine is much easier than choosing healthier foods," she says. "If someone is still eating Big Macs every day, and then [works out] three times a week, the weight will come off quickly at first, but eventually a plateau will be reached and the weight loss will cease. That leads to frustration and eventually folks give up a fitness plan altogether."

Of course not every woman is comfortable sweating or

getting physical. I was a rough and tumble tomboy growing up, playing kickball, volleyball, basketball, and baseball, and I still enjoy sports to this day. Cathy, on the other hand, was content to stay in the house, do her nails, sew her own outfits, record soap operas on the reel-to-reel, and plan her next party.

Some women who have tried going to gyms wonder why the "skinny Mini's" who populate many health clubs are even there in the first place. For an overweight or obese woman, being around all those buff bodies can be intimidating, making her feel like all eyes are on her. So she decides not to go at all.

But exercise does not have to be excruciating and can take many forms that are actually fun. Donna Richardson's friendly and inspiring "Sweating in the Spirit" is an excellent workout video for beginners. It allows you to exercise at your own pace in the privacy of your living room.

Beginning line dancing and water aerobics (great for seniors) offer cheap, good workouts and are taught at many community centers. Women's self-defense classes are also available through parks and recreation departments and at local YWCAs. The Black Ski Club has been around for years, with chapters in every major city, and offers a fun way to stay fit by hitting the slopes during the winter and hosting gatherings throughout the year.

Whatever you choose, it's important to get moving. It has been proven that people who exercise regularly, regardless of the method they choose, not only stay in better physical condition, but also enjoy an improved emotional and mental outlook.

The Trouble with Hair

Hair and working out may seem unrelated to those outside the black community, but sisters know only too well how to avoid "messin' up our hair." Some women simply will not work out on a regular basis because of the trauma (a burnout perm) and drama ("will the new beautician do a good job?") of maintaining beautiful, manageable, straight hair. Touch-ups, nappy roots, and "kitchens" are facts of life for black women. The texture of our hair, which "goes back," or reverts to its natural state with sweat or moisture, means making regular visits to the hairdresser. And these appointments are as important as putting gas in our cars. Because of the designs we like and our other unique hair-care needs, keeping it straight can be a lot more complicated, not to mention a lot more expensive, than simply applying over-the-counter hair goods.

One coed told me, "I can't afford to sweat out a press every week, and I don't have the time to get it done on the regular." At forty bucks a pop, a weekly press-and-curl to straighten hair can be expensive. For middle-class working black women who like wearing their hair straightened, it's a question of time more than money, sandwiching lengthy, frequent hair appointments in between jobs and family obligations. Or, depending on where we live, sometimes it's difficult to find a quality hairdresser we can trust with our tresses. For these and other reasons, many women forgo regular exercise to keep their hair looking good.

One sister took extreme measures. "I had to cut mine all off," says Loni, an African American college administrator who sports a close-cropped 'fro and is committed to being physically fit by jogging and playing golf. Loni resides in a predominately white neighborhood and says not only are black hair-care products not available within close range of her home, but the nearest black hairdresser is also a distance. To save time and aggravation, she gave up wearing her hair straight through presses and perms and keeps her hair short.

The African American female is taught from early in life that hair is not only her "crowing glory," but also her validation in a world obsessed with the outer self. Around the time we outgrow hopscotch and double Dutch we also want to get rid of girlish plaits and barrettes, and adopt more grown-up (straight) hairstyles.

Since back when we discovered chitlins, the length and texture of black hair have been a source of classism, political identity, and mainstream acceptance. As slaves, black women covered their hair with "do-rags," cut it off, or wore plaits while working the fields. However, when a white slave-owner fathered a child by a black woman, that newborn's hair often was more straight than nappy. Thus, Caucasian-type hair gradually came to be considered "good" hair (as in white) while tresses that were naturally tightly curled or "nappy" were labeled "bad."

Unfortunately this kind of thinking still exists in the black community, influenced not only by intraracial prejudices but also by the Eurocentric mass media that equates beauty with looking white. As a result, many black women press, perm, or weave their hair straight in order to be considered attractive and conventional.

Black women who work out regularly tend to opt for natural

styles, braids, wigs, twists, and dreadlocks—which are perfectly fine if you own your own business or work in education, the arts, or other professions that require less conformity. However, in corporate America, those who fit into the company culture are considered valuable employees. Black women working in a conservative environment may be less inclined to risk rocking the boat by wearing their hair naturally, which might be considered too Afrocentric for a company's image. Blending in without drawing attention to your hair—no matter how qualified you are—could mean a promotion or a raise in pay. Even today, cornrows and French braids raise eyebrows in some quarters and are considered unprofessional.

The urgent health crisis, however, begs the question: Does a black woman have to choose between being in shape and looking beautiful? Faced with the current obesity predicament, isn't it time we viewed things through a different lens, adopting a new vision of beauty for African Americans and all women that relies less on superficiality and more on physical and emotional well-being? Being healthy—whether thin or full-figured, nappy or straight—means loving and accepting who we are, while reaching for improvement and happily resisting an arbitrary standard of beauty imposed on us by others.

Califia Dreamin'

When we ponder the physical allure of the African American woman, superstars who light up the screen like Queen Latifah, women who strut like Tyra, and sisters who can shake that thang like Janet come to mind. But as legend has it, one Amazon-like woman so captivated the heart of a famous man, he named his newly discovered territory for her.

Her name was Queen Califia, leader of a population that sixteenth-century Spanish explorer Hernando Cortés described as consisting of "big black women with strong and passionate hearts and great virtues," who lived north of Baja.[5] So enthralled was Cortés by the inhabitants of this island utopia and by Queen Califia that he named the newly explored territory "California" in her honor. Some African American researchers who have studied the history of the Golden State say the state's name literally translates to "where black women live."

But much like the biblical Lilith, Califia is not found in most history books and her story is refuted by many scholars, who dismiss it as being as unreliable as that of the two-headed beasts that Cortés also recorded in his diaries.

Today, mythological Queen Califia is the subject of paintings, books, and poetry, as both Hispanics and African Americans claim her as their own. For black women in particular, Califia is empowering because her physicality mesmerized the rugged Cortés. Even as myth, Califia represents a symbol of guile and beauty, one of the few positive role models from yesterday for today's young girls of color. Not many of us will have a state named for us, but plus-size women, like all women, can beguile and challenge men.

Rob's Recommendations

Tenderheaded: A Comb-Bending Collection of Hair Stories, edited by Pamela Johnson and Juliette Harris, introduction by Ntozake Shange; published by Washington Square Press, 2002.

I AM: A Poetic Journey Towards Self Definition, by Stephanie Pruitt, published by Infotainment Talent and Publishing, 2002.

Kindred, by Octavia Butler, published by Beacon Press, 1979, reissued 2004. The story of a contemporary African American woman transported in time to a slave plantation in the South. A scary good read.

Hollywood's Finest

Roots. A classic television miniseries based on the book by Alex Haley. On video and DVD. 1976.

School Daze. A Spike Lee film about "jigaboos and wannabes," class struggles and intra-racial prejudice. 1988.

CHAPTER THREE

Can a Big Sister Get Some Love?

She is too educated, too strong, too successful,
too stubborn and too hard to control.

— Former husband of large and in-charge WANGARI MAATHAI,
world-renowned environmentalist and 2004 Nobel
Peace Prize winner from Kenya

"BE NICE TO HIM . . . ."

That's what Cathy whispered to me when she first introduced her husband, Luke, to the family. At age thirty-six, Cathy had never dated a lot, and when she met Luke at the bank where they both worked, she fell hard.

We accepted Luke because Cathy was madly in love with him. But I guess no man would have been good enough for my sister. Though he worked hard for years at the job my father got him at the Los Angeles County Sanitation District, Luke was as helpless at home as one of the babies Cathy cared for. Other than the money he needed for cigarettes and gas, Luke signed over his paycheck and the managing of the household to my sister. "Cathy did everything for him," laughs Lynn, Cathy's former boss and one of her closest friends. "Luke did not even know how to make toast."

A petite, flush-faced man with prematurely white hair, Luke was just a few years older than Cathy and had been married three times before. He had a number of children from other relationships; some he was in contact with, others he was not. People assumed because Luke is white, their interracial marriage put Cathy under extra pressure to be thin and conform to a Eurocentric perception of beauty. No one from the outside looking in ever really knows what goes on in a marriage. I can say, however, that neither I nor friends and family ever remember hearing Luke make fun of her weight. "Cathy was heavy when the two of them met," says Theresa, our sister, "and he loved Cathy for who she was. Cathy's weight issues were inside her own head."

In fact the only times when Cathy was not worried about her weight was when she was planning her weddings — all three of them to Luke. Decked out in sweeping size-26 gowns, with yards of lace trailing behind, Cathy turned into a stunning bride during each of her "re-commitment" ceremonies. The thrice-repeated matrimonies were Cathy's time to be queen for a day with all her fans (i.e., friends and family) on hand to feed her fantasy of a happily-ever-after marriage to Luke, her skinny prince in a rented tux. "I just loved being married," Cathy laughed.

However, not long before she died, Luke and Cathy temporarily separated and Luke moved in with another woman. While they were apart, Cathy's spur-of-the-moment celebrations were fewer, the ring in my sister's laugh a bit dimmer. She was consumed with dreaming up ways to get Luke back home. He eventually did return. But in hindsight I think Cathy's rush to surgery, shortly after their reconciliation, was a kind of matrimonial insurance in case her husband decided to go missing in action again. Cathy was hoping for a brand new body and a marriage reborn.

Her friend Lynn puts it this way: "Oh, Luke probably did not say in so many words, 'Yes, have the surgery,' once he got wind of Cathy's plans . . . it was probably more like, 'Well, if you think it will help you to be healthy . . .'"

All in the Family

Millions of plus-size women of all races enjoy healthy, happy, long-term marriages. The idea of weight-loss surgery is the furthest thing from their minds. Nearly half of all African American women are married, according to the U.S. Census Bureau, and countless others live within committed relationships. My younger sister Sheilah Wilks, a full-figured hospice worker, has been married to her husband, William, for nearly twenty-seven years. Such unions in the African American community never make headlines or are featured topics on talk shows.

But extra weight can put a strain on a relationship. Some women are overweight when they marry; others become "fat and happy" in the years after "jumping the broom." Then there's the weight gain that comes with childbearing and from aging. The lifestyle choices of married African Americans are also a factor. A

2004 Centers for Disease Control study found that black married couples are less physically active than single, divorced, and widowed people; and, not surprisingly, more black husbands and wives are overweight and obese than are African Americans who have never married, or are widowed or living with a partner.[1]

Despite the cultural factors that can contribute to a woman's weight problems, some women feel enormous pressure and prejudice from both inside and outside the home. A husband who years ago married a slender bride may feel "tricked" by his now-overweight wife — even if his waistline has also expanded with time. One woman told me she hates to look at "the skinny girl" in her wedding photos and covers her face whenever a camera is pointed her way. A few women admitted they feel ashamed of their heavier bodies and have lost interest in having sex now that they have put on extra pounds.

Forget about trying to maneuver into creative love-making positions, laughed one middle-aged African American wife who struggles with her weight and suffers from high blood pressure: "These days, I get tired and out of breath when I'm in bed with my husband."

Weight problems may have a detrimental effect on a marriage, as well as on an entire family. Women often talk about how difficult it is to change eating habits and exercise regularly. As discussed in Chapter Two, lots of families are used to eating fattening home-cooked meals or going to Mickey D's or ordering pizza for dinner. Exchanging Big Macs for green salads and broiled chicken breasts may not go over well. Leisure time in many black families is spent in front of the television, playing cards or dominos, or surfing the Net, rather than engaging in sports or other physical activities.

Sometimes there's camaraderie in overeating. "My husband is my 'snacking buddy,' and he always sabotages me whenever I try to diet," one stay-at-home mom reveals. Vanessa, a U.S. postal worker, watched her boyfriend grow so threatened by the idea that she was about to become a slimmer mate, he cursed her mere hours before she was scheduled to have a gastric bypass. "He told me, 'I hope you die on the operating table,'" Vanessa recalls. She came through the surgery fine, dropped the excess weight, and lost the boyfriend.

Even though being overweight does not automatically mean a woman is in poor health, carrying extra pounds often can lead to physical dangers. When diabetes or hypertension hits home, weight becomes a critical issue that affects the entire household. The whole family may have to adjust to Mom's new aches and pains, stress headaches and fatigue, her short temper and high anxiety, frequent doctor's appointments, money spent on new medications, revolving diets, swearing off salt and sweets, and trying to remain positive in the face of a serious health concern.

Sticks and Stones May Break My Bones . . .

Negative stereotypes about the sexual desirability of large black women abound. I will never forget the time I was giving a lecture, entitled "From Auction Block to Idiot Box," on the image of African American women in popular culture. I began by asking the audience at California State University, Fullerton, to tell me the first thing that comes to mind when they think of the black woman.

Overwhelmingly, the response was someone who is "strong." When I asked them to come up with another adjective, most in the room exchanged puzzled looks, but one young man in the back had his answer ready.

"Black women are fat and angry," he hollered. The room was stunned. "They're mad because black men are dating white women," he continued. "African American women are so fat, no one wants to date them."

Some outraged young women in the audience joined me in asking the man what survey he had done to determine such nonsense. "I heard it on Tom Leykis," the young man said proudly, referring to the radio shock-jock who broadcasts his sexist rants to millions of impressionable young men on a daily basis. I responded that the tendency to paint countless black women with one broad brush is an example of the destructive "idiot box" mentality.

Truth be told, the young man was simply repeating common misconceptions about the lovability of big black women, especially among those whose only knowledge of African Americans is gleaned from the evening news, movies, or TV. Demeaning attitudes are realities plus-size black women face every day. Folks assume because a woman is overweight, she is also lazy, bossy, lacking in personal hygiene and ambition, oversexed or asexual, and unmoved by ugly stereotyping.

Many overweight women I spoke to professed pride in their lives and their appearance despite the gawking, the insults, and the constant fat prejudice. This self-affirming attitude serves as a psychic armor in a fat-phobic world. Others use an outwardly confident attitude to mask the shame and helplessness they feel because of their weight. Valinda, a plus-size philosophy major, says she hangs on to her "extra padding" as a way to avoid sex. "Not intentionally, of course," she admits. "It's just when you have *the* man or different men coming on to you a lot, a way of discouraging so much sexual attention is to put on weight. . . . Other than that, food is damn good."

Stephanie, a thirty-three-year-old single parent and part-time college student, used to describe herself as "super-sized" when she weighed over three hundred pounds before weight-loss surgery. She remembers feeling both conspicuous and invisible when it came to the opposite sex.

Etched in Stephanie's mind is an incident in an L.A. highrise. A professionally dressed black man got on the elevator with Stephanie and never made eye contact. Instead, remembers Stephanie, the atmosphere was tense, and the guy kept his gaze glued to the floor until the doors opened and he bolted out.

"I could write a book all about how black men treat fat women," Stephanie proclaims. "I will never forget that time in the elevator. I wanted to shout at him, 'Speak to a sista, will you? I am still your sister whether or not I am fat.'" After weight-loss surgery, she lost one hundred and fifty pounds in just over two years. She did it because, even though she enjoyed healthy relationships with many men, some men reacted to her in a negative way. "[Before I lost the weight] they started treating me like 'the fat girl'—a person who did not matter, who needn't be acknowledged or spoken to, someone who was less than a human being."

Typically upbeat and cheerful, Stephanie's voice lowers with hurt and rage when she recalls the black men who ignored her and treated her like she was "nothing" when she was fat. "Black men would not even extend to me common courtesies, like holding the door open." Stephanie insists that white and Hispanic men were more likely to look her in the eye and acknowledge her than was a black man. "If you are physically unappealing to a black man in any way," Stephanie believes, "some act like you don't even exist."

One Size Fits All?

"No one wants a bone but a dog" is an old saying in the black community that affirms the traditional approval of full-figured women by black men. But attitudes may be changing. Being overweight can be dangerous to your health and also stigmatizing, as Stephanie experienced. The long-standing perception that sisters are "satisfied" with being overweight or obese—and that black men like them that way—has led society in general to discount the medical dangers that can accompany weight problems. (That black women's health issues are marginalized and ignored overall was front and center before millions of television viewers during the

2004 Vice Presidential debates. Both Vice President Dick Cheney and Senator John Edwards were asked what they would do about the fact that black women are becoming infected with HIV/AIDS at alarming rates. The men expressed surprise about the crisis. I can only imagine what they would have said — or not said — about black women and the problem of obesity.)

Body-type preferences are no longer easily defined. Young African American men who are products of the middle class are inclined to adopt more mainstream American values, including a preference for a thinner woman. A January 2004 study published in the *Journal of Black Studies* reported that African American men between the ages of eighteen and thirty-five attending predominantly white colleges in the southeastern United States found smaller women more attractive than women with larger body types.[2]

Couple this with the white standard of beauty screaming at us from MTV, BET, and other media sources, and it's no wonder outlooks are changing among young African American men and women alike.

This could explain why the average sister who has weight-loss surgery is just thirty-nine years old. These women have come of age with music videos, twenty-four-seven cable channels, and the World Wide Web. With this media frenzy has come the revival of an age-old stereotype of the black woman as "she-devil." Dr. Gail Wyatt, a leading expert on black sexuality, describes this sister as an "immoral, conniving seductress who loves sex anytime, anywhere. . . ."[3]

The hyperactive, booty-bouncing sister, portrayed as a love cheat and skank in popular video culture, is really just a modern-day resurrection of the she-devil, the black temptress who gets what is coming to her.

Crystal Crawford is director of public policy for the California Black Women's Health Project, which studies African American women's health concerns. Crawford believes that although the black community has traditionally been more accepting of a larger body type, "Some women recently want to look like Halle [Berry]. We as black people don't necessarily admire people who are emaciated; however, when folks are one hundred pounds over-weight or more, there becomes a kind of diminishing returns," in addition to the potential for serious health consequences.

Crawford sees the increasing popularity of liposuction and weight-loss surgeries with urban and suburban black women as a sign that sisters are rejecting the "Big Mama" character-ization—the sexless mistress of the kitchen—that has been with us since the days of slavery. "Today, women are willing to go to extremes to find a quick fix as a way of getting that male attention," Crawford says. "Black women want to be perceived as so-called 'cute and small.' Society says that 'petite' is what is beau-tiful. We as black people have always embraced fuller figures. But nowadays, the media images are working on us in the sense that more and more black women desire to be thin."

Regardless of whether a woman has been fat her entire life or has gained the "college twenty, thirty, forty, or fifty," the women I interviewed in writing this book who view weight as a "major personal issue," expressed more dissatisfaction with the social consequences—demoralizing experiences with men and fat discrimination—than with critical physical concerns associated with obesity. Some recall having been taunted or ignored by men because of their physiques, while at the same time being assured by well-meaning family members that "you're fine just the way you are" and that black men "like big women."

For some women, loss of love leads them to take desperate measures to lose weight. Terri, a thirty-year-old from Houston who works in the health-care field, yearned for a makeover—something, anything to ease the pain—after she broke up with her cheating fiancé. She considered weight-loss surgery but could only afford liposuction. She describes how her attempts to pay back her wayward boyfriend could have landed her behind bars: "I was about twenty-four years old, and my fiancé and I broke up because he was cheating on me. Although he denied it, I left him and he ended up marrying the other woman."

Terri's shock turned to unbridled fury—and a campaign for revenge. "I did everything from sabotage his college degree (he had forged his transcript from a previous college, so I informed his current college, which got him in *deep* trouble). I got him fired from his job. I stalked him by phone and in person. I put sugar in his gas tank. After all that, I still felt ugly. I started to re-evaluate myself and went into a deep depression."

Turning her anger on herself, Terri decided to go under the knife. "I considered weight-loss surgery and a nose job. I could not afford either. But I had my financial aid check and I discovered I could afford liposuction. I went into debt to get the surgery and used all of my school loan money. After the surgery and healing, I still felt useless and horrible. I still felt ugly and depressed. It took me a long time to realize that it wasn't my appearance I needed to alter; it was my inside — how I felt about myself."

Eventually Terri found self-acceptance and a way to forgive. "The surgery took away the fat but not the internal pain. A lot of the fat came back anyway. I stopped comparing myself to others and worked on myself inside and out. I tried to work on dysfunctional relationships with my friends and family and my spirituality. I even apologized to my ex for all the stuff I did to retaliate against him. It made me feel good when he apologized (somewhat) to me and even tried to get back with me. I doubt if I would go under the knife again — at least not for the wrong reasons."

Men in Search of Queen-Size Love

Despite her negative experiences, like with the guy on the elevator, Stephanie reports that she has enjoyed positive dating relationships, including one with a well-to-do African American real estate entrepreneur. "I have known Michael for years and he treats me like a queen," Stephanie says. "He tells me all the time he liked my body better when I weighed one hundred and fifty pound more. He thinks I am too small now."

"The men I meet adore me, my body," says Elizabeth, a plus-size graphic artist. "They'll say things like, 'I like being with you because there is more to hold on to,' and 'You're soft and cushy.' I think some men see a woman with big breasts and imagine a cushion, a place they can bury their face and feel safe."

An executive booking manager for a Los Angeles–area speakers' bureau, Juanita describes herself as large and lovely and "a player in the dating scene." She does not see herself as anyone's wife — ever. "There are lots of men who like me because I am a big woman," Juanita says. "I have never had a problem with men not liking me because of my weight; my personality shines. And men always comment on my pretty eyes. Obviously they admire the essence of me. They also like my other body parts too."

Tina, a diminutive, thirty-eight-year-old African American woman who has dated both men and women for the past twelve years, says that guys are usually "looking for a woman who is smaller in size than they are, and women typically look for taller men. With lesbians, though, a woman's shape and height are usually not that important." Tina does believe, though, that even within the gay community large women are often misjudged. "When I see a big woman at the clubs, I assume she is a 'stud' — more stereotypically masculine than feminine — but that is not always true."

It's true that some men prefer big women and choose them in the same way others favor blonds. Anecdotally speaking, a voluptuous woman could represent the ideal mother/lover image for some men. Ron, a fifty-three-year-old special education teacher, told me he never dates a woman "under a size 12" who has "food issues" and "does not like to eat."

Many men associate a woman who has a passion for food with someone who is highly sexual and likes to cook. Other guys admit to being attracted to the body type they are most familiar with from their big-boned and fleshy sisters and mother. This can explain why some African American women are miffed when they see their favorite black movie star or NBA idol photographed with a woman who has a "flat chest and no ass."

Jerome, a middle-aged African American grocery clerk who has dated large women his entire life, buys into the notion that "big women are easier. They don't expect much and if they reject a brother, he does not feel as bad as if a skinny woman disses him." Besides, Jerome says that in his experience "little women are evil."

Hidden agendas and self-hate can create emotional land-mines in any intimate relationship. And, according to Stephanie, there is a world of difference between a man who loves and appreciates big women and so-called "chubby chasers." The latter are men with a fetish, obsessed with fatty flesh. Elizabeth, the graphic designer, calls such men "vultures who find and exploit [a woman] they think may have low self-esteem because of her size. Chubby chasers really don't like themselves and come to us figuring we must also feel bad about ourselves too. They think we'll be a perfect match."

Stephanie agrees. "Chasers are losers . . . especially the guys who troll the Internet chat rooms and place personal ads. Those are the kinds of guys who are really looking for vulnerable women to play 'mama' to them."

Chubby chasers may be desperately seeking women to support them and forgive them their infidelities and other faults in the same way that they might seek approval from an understanding parent. Chubby chasers are often in search of a woman with a big body and a big heart to match. Stephanie remembers encountering lots of men during her super-sized days who were "closet chubby chasers" — guys who wanted to be seen in public with a slender girl, but when they got home, they wanted to "do it" with an obese or overweight woman.

You don't have to be overweight to attract a jerk, like a chubby chaser. To paraphrase spiritualist and author Marianne Williamson's book, *A Return to Love*, it's one thing to attract a silver-tongued devil; it's another thing to give him your phone number.

No matter your size, there are going to be challenges in your love life. If you feel overwhelmed (or underwhelmed) by the love in your life, here are some "Rob-isms" to take to heart:

- You deserve to be loved unconditionally and respected regardless of your weight. There are plenty of men who appreciate big women and will treat you like a queen.

- A chubby chaser is a man more interested in the size of your dresses and pocketbook than in your capacity for love. He is not worthy of you. If he tells you, "I like big women," take it as a compliment — just make sure that's not all he likes about you. Beware a man who consistently tries to sabotage your efforts to lose weight and encourages unhealthy eating. If he persists in bringing donuts around when you are counting calories, you could grit your teeth and fight temptation. Or you could drop him like a bad habit.

- On the other hand, be suspect of any man who puts undue pressure on you to lose weight. If he suggests that you will "look better" or he hints that he's "concerned about your health," these comments may be born from genuine love and caring, or they may signal his creeping dissatisfaction with your weight. Ask yourself, if you were fat when he met you, what right does he have to try and change you now? If you try to lose weight for someone else, your efforts will likely result in frustration and failure — or in taking potentially life-threatening risks. If you desire long-term weight loss, see a doctor or nutritionist or join a support group to help you get started. Remember there's a fine line between encouraging and manipulating. There's an even finer line between someone who says, "I respect your choices," and someone who says, "Do whatever you damn well please."

- Just because you always look good on the outside — your hair is whipped, your makeup is perfect, and you sport the latest designer fashions — does not mean that carrying too much weight will not cause you serious health problems down the road. If you want to lose weight, do it for yourself, but don't be afraid to get professional assistance in choosing a plan that works for you.

- Society, with its relentless media images featuring mostly thin women as beautiful and desirable, has conditioned us to be biased against and disdainful of fat people. *Do not* accept this as *your* truth. Every human being deserves to be treated with respect and dignity. There are many worse things than being overweight — like being fat-phobic and narrow-minded.

Rob's Recommendations

The Beauty Myth: How Images of Beauty Are Used Against Women, by Naomi Wolf, published by William Morrow, 1991.

Black and Single: Meeting and Choosing a Partner Who's Right for You, by Dr. Larry Davis, published by Noble Press, 1993.

The Best Kind of Loving: A Black Woman's Guide to Finding Intimacy, by Gwendolyn Goldsby Grant, published by HarperCollins, 1995.

How to Love a Black Woman, by Ronn Elmore, published by Warner Books, 1999.

What Brothers Think, What Sistahs Know: The Real Deal on Love and Relationships, by husband and wife team Denene Millner and Nick Chiles, published by William Morrow and Company, 1999.

Hollywood's Finest

Diary of a Mad Black Woman. Starring Kimberly Elise and Tyler Perry as Madea. 2005.

Big Mama's House. Comedy starring Martin Lawrence in drag. 2000.

Hoodlum. With Loretta Devine and Queen Latifah. 1997.

Soul Food. "Big Mama" casts her wise shadow over her troubled yet loving family. 1997.

CHAPTER FOUR

Digging Our Graves
with Our Forks

*There are times when I have to hurt through a situation,
and when this happens, the choice is not whether to hurt or
not to hurt, but what to do while I am hurting.*
—ANONYMOUS member of a twelve-step program

CATHY HAD FUNNY eating habits. She could starve herself all
day long, sipping only Diet Coke from the huge thermos she kept
within arm's reach. Come midnight when the house was asleep,
she wanted not just a bedtime snack, but her first full-on meal of
the day. I remember how she savored a well-done T-bone steak,
macaroni and cheese from the box, baked ham, and maybe a
glass of burgundy, chuckling as the guilty party broke down on
late-night *Perry Mason*.

Sometimes she had food cravings that lasted for weeks. Our
sister Theresa recalls Cathy coming to visit her in Minneapolis.
From the time Cathy arrived, she pined for Mexican food. "Of
course there are plenty of Mexican food restaurants here," Theresa

says. "But for some reason they weren't good enough. The whole time she was here she complained that she needed Mexican food. Before she flew back to California, she called some friends and insisted they meet her at LAX with Mexican food from her favorite restaurant."

Back in the 1960s when we were teenagers, in the days of Jack LaLanne, before America turned into a diet-crazed nation, Cathy was the only person I knew who obsessed over her weight and what she ate. Forever counting calories and yelling at the scale, Cathy — the middle of seven children — was always the center of attention. You could take our family's temperature by Cathy's moods: If she was happy and planning a party, the whole family prepared to celebrate; if she was depressed or anxious, we felt her pain. I don't recall Cathy being a particularly big eater, however (although she could eat Ruffles with blue cheese dip and Snickers until the sun came up). She did not eat often during the day, but her favorite foods were sugar-laden and high in fat. And like many working mothers, Cathy seemed to enjoy her food most when she ate alone.

Elizabeth, the graphic artist, says she relates to Cathy's eating choices. "I can only imagine what people are thinking when they see me walking down the street because I am so overweight," she says. "The CIA could get out their best lie detector test and give it to me and people would know that I don't eat as much as it looks like I do. I only eat one or two meals a day at the most." She later admits, "I even criticize other fat people, thinking, 'Why is that person eating at McDonald's?' I have to catch myself, because I have no idea what they are going through and they probably don't sit at the table and eat all day to get to the size they are."

When Cathy moved out of our parents' home, her weight worries went with her. She began working full time, and took regular trips with a group of her pals to Tijuana, Mexico, to receive shots that were supposed to suppress her appetite so she could lose weight. Neither Mexican shots nor diet pills worked for long. Her dissatisfaction with her weight and body continued until the day she died.

As I try to reconstruct my sister's motivations, I still cannot understand why Cathy was so negative about her appearance that she was willing to risk her life to alter herself. I suppose no one really knows what anguish lives in the soul of another, even a sister whom you've loved your entire life.

"Cathy was codependent," Theresa says. "She was kind and loving with a big heart, always there for everyone, listening to their problems, trying to help them out. Just look at the dysfunctional people who were always around her." Theresa refers to the revolving door of needy friends and acquaintances who were part of Cathy's everyday life. "We were Cathy's kinfolk, but they were really her family."

I used to reject the notion that a group of strangers could be closer to my sister than her own blood. But in hindsight I see the truth in that dynamic. Cathy's open heart and generosity were magnets for the dependent personalities who clung to her. Yet even her collection of close-knit relationships could not erase the gloom beneath her radiant smile.

Several years before her surgery, the tension in Cathy's life escalated. She decided to move her in-home daycare business to a separate location; but when the bills became too overwhelming, she moved the business back home, feeling as though she had failed miserably. Then Luke moved out. And Cathy started the hunt for a permanent solution to what she felt was her most serious problem — her weight.

Eating the Blues Away

Even though Cathy was never officially diagnosed, I believe part of her negative self-image stemmed from untreated depression. She saw a therapist for a while when she was in her twenties, but she was never told she suffered from a medical condition other than hypertension. Millions of black women who experience depression, which can manifest itself in distorted eating habits, remain undiagnosed and untreated.

According to the National Health Association, a person who is depressed may experience reduced appetite and weight loss, increased appetite and weight gain, or persistent physical problems, such as chronic pain or digestive disorders that do not respond to treatment.

In addition, regular indulgence in so-called "comfort foods" — chocolate, potato chips, our favorite caffeine drinks from Starbucks, and sugary sodas — as a way of dealing with boredom or anxiety can end up worsening the problem by creating headaches and mood swings. "Jonesing" for a cheeseburger and a Coke is the body's response to the addictive components like casomorphins in cheese and refined sugars in breads and other starchy foods that give you a temporary high before the inevitable late-afternoon meltdown.

Black women are not unique in using food to escape the blues. Lots of women reach for the chips or pop M&Ms to temporarily feel better. A trained professional can help us become aware of our eating patterns and find ways to better cope with life's ups and downs. According to the National Institute of Mental Health, depression is usually accompanied by one or more of the following symptoms:

- Constantly feeling sad, anxious, or in an "empty" mood.
- Sleeping too much or too little, or waking up in the middle of the night or early morning.
- Loss of pleasure and interest in sex.
- Restlessness, irritability.
- Difficulty concentrating or remembering, feeling fatigued.
- Feeling guilty, hopeless, or worthless, and imagining scenarios in which you are taking your own life.

The Office of the Surgeon General of the United States estimates 17 million people suffer from clinical depression. Most women across ethnicities experience depression at some point in their lives, and African American and Hispanic women are twice as likely as men to be depressed. Ongoing depression can result from many things: racism, unemployment, incarceration, relationships, careers, higher incidence of poverty, and reproductive events including the menstrual cycle, pregnancy, postpartum, infertility, menopause, or the decision not to have children.

The good news is that 80 percent of the folks suffering from depression can be successfully treated with psychotherapy or medication. If you suffer over an extended period of time from any symptoms mentioned above, you should seek help immediately.

Unfortunately, the medical community at large doesn't always respond appropriately to the needs of black people. In the case of depression, African Americans are often misdiagnosed or treated only with antidepressants instead of a combination of medication and psychotherapy, which could help us gain self-awareness and perhaps have more control over circumstances that might be contributing to the depression. On the other hand, some black women may feel better privately taking a pill rather than risk their loved ones finding out that they've seen a shrink. Regardless of the treatment, it is critical that people who are medically depressed seek and receive the proper long-term help.

Do We Love Our Bodies?

Dr. Price Cobbs is the coauthor of *Black Rage*, written in 1968 and widely acclaimed as the first book to examine black life from the vantage point of psychiatry and the insidious effects of the heritage of slavery. He believes that some black women gain weight as a "reaction to the excess attention that black women's sexuality attracts. . . ."[1] For example, during the time of slavery, black women had little control over their own bodies. Our foremothers were routinely raped by slave masters, impregnated, and forced to bear children from their rapists. A psychic disconnect developed about our bodies that even today makes some black women feel separated from their sexuality and physical being.

Dr. Cobbs believes black people to some extent have been encouraged by the majority community to tolerate obesity, which I believe is a subtle form of racism and what some call "the bigotry of low expectations." Dr. Cobbs says, "African Americans wind up accepting things we should not be accepting." With 70 percent of African American women now considered overweight or obese, Dr. Cobbs's theory from nearly forty years ago is no longer entirely accurate.

Elizabeth started gaining weight in high school, and laughs that "my big hips come from my dad's side because my mother is extremely small." Elizabeth, who never knew her father, regularly braves the dating scene but says she knows lots of overweight women who don't dare: Some sisters "hold on to extra weight as physical and psychological protection against a hostile world. The thinking goes like this: If I am fat already, I don't have to concern myself about going out and trying to find a man, because I already know that most men want thin women. So many women think, 'Oh my God, if I lost weight, someone might actually be attracted to me and I might have a relationship—and risk being rejected for some other reason.'"

Beyond the immediate issue of using excess weight to avoid intimacy lurks another tragedy for some women. They turn to food to ease the painful memories of childhood sexual abuse. Sadly, young women and girls who've been molested, often by a relative or close family friend—someone they knew and trusted—grow up harboring the secret and the shame, attempting to bury them through various forms of addiction.

Farlane, an alcohol and drug counselor with a master's degree in psychology, has fought addiction demons much of her adult life. As a child, she lived next door to three older children who molested Yvette for years. She believes that nightmare contributed to her never-ending battle with her weight.

Before her gastric bypass, Virginia, a single mother of four, spent years in therapy trying to come to terms with the fact that her biological father forced her to have sex with him throughout her teenage years. Memories still haunt Virginia to the point that to this day she cannot even speak her father's name.

Elizabeth says she too was molested as a child, but she does not make the connection between childhood sexual abuse and obesity. "Yes, I was molested by a family member as a child," Elizabeth reveals. "But that is not the reason I am overweight. I am overweight because it is in my genes to be fat, because I was thin as a child."

Robin Stone's book, *No Secrets, No Lies: How Black Families Can Heal from Sexual Abuse*, is described as "an honest and illuminating look at the soul-shattering effects of sexual abuse." It lists eating disorders as one of the most common "psychological, emotional, and behavioral effects of sexual abuse."[2]

Sex abuse experts say some victims of incest use overeating to escape inner turmoil and downplay their femininity, avoiding unwanted attention to their bodies by wearing baggy clothes or gaining too much weight.

According to literature published by Survivors of Incest Anonymous, "If we perceive obesity to be unattractive, and if we believe we were abused because we were attractive, we may overeat in a misguided attempt to defend ourselves from further sexual assault."[3] Some large black women mistakenly believe that their size can protect them from physical assaults, including rape. This is not true. Any woman can be vulnerable to a date rape or other attack.

In his twenty-five years of treating obesity, Dr. Michael Myers, a weight-loss specialist in Los Alamitos, California, concludes that 40 percent of his patients have been victims of childhood sexual abuse. "There is some experimental evidence that suggests increases in so-called 'stress hormones,' such as cortisol, that result from extreme psychological stress can induce the proliferation of fat cells and predispose sexual abuse victims to the development of obesity."

Myers began writing about this phenomenon decades ago, and more recently other sociologists and psychologists have published similar findings that address the link between sexual abuse and obesity. "It has been known for years that sexual abuse of women is associated with eating disorders like anorexia nervosa and bulimia nervosa," says Dr. Myers. Many adults are surprised to learn that black girls today suffer from anorexia nervosa (called "ana" among teen sufferers), the psycho-physiological disorder characterized by an abnormal fear of becoming obese, a distorted self-image, a persistent unwillingness to eat, and severe weight loss sometimes accompanied by self-induced vomiting, excessive exercise, and malnutrition. Bulimia (also known as "mia"), an eating disorder characterized by guilt, depression, self-condemnation, binging, and later vomiting, is another ailment appearing increasingly in the African American community.

Dr. Myers goes on to say, "But now many of the physicians who treat obesity believe there also exists a strong correlation between sexual abuse and the onset of adult obesity."

In a sense, obesity protects people from their sexuality since in Western culture obese people are not generally perceived as sexually desirable. Dr. Myers finds that survivors of sexual abuse have low self-esteem and severe problems with depression, often feeling that it was their fault they were sexually abused — "an emotional but totally illogical belief."

Dr. Susan Fellows, professor of sociology, believes that if sexual abuse is not dealt with, it can result in self-destructiveness in the form of "dis-eases," like drug and alcohol addiction, overeating, and suicide. Dr. Fellows has studied eating disorders and believes people who try to deal with childhood trauma through therapy and attempt to change their lives are often sabotaged by their families and loved ones. This doesn't always happen deliberately, but any change in one family member "rocks the boat" for the others. "For example," she says, "for a man to say that he would prefer his partner dead rather than for her to lose weight is obviously an emotional and mental abuser. . . . The speaker is scared of losing some sort of power in the relationship."

Dr. Fellows believes "it is important that treatment for sexual abuse and obesity includes recovery for the whole family or at least a few significant others." Eating disorders resulting in obesity are like drug abuse. They're public health problems, not moral failings. The solutions to both problems, according to Dr. Fellows, are promoting health education and nurturing self-esteem.

Help is available for women who suffer from overeating and other disorders related to childhood sexual abuse. The Veterans Administration (VA) lists childhood sexual abuse (CSA) as a condition that can bring about post-traumatic stress disorder (PTSD). Veterans and their families are eligible to receive treatment through educational classes available from a local VA center. Counseling through Sexaholics Anonymous and Survivors of Incest Anonymous is free, and groups such as the Rape, Abuse and Incest National Network offer twenty-four-hour crisis intervention online and in person.

Speak for Yourself

The first step to emotional health is honesty with self, family, and professionals who can help. We must ask ourselves, What is our relationship with food and how do we really feel about our bodies? Is food our best friend or a dreaded enemy? Discussions of weight and dieting inspire feelings of guilt and remorse for lots of people. Many simply want to deny the problem of obesity, acknowledging that we may be overweight and obese, but seeing no need to talk about it.

As females, we are taught it's rude to comment on a woman's weight and size (to her face), that those are personal matters that need not be discussed. Black women who don't know wrinkles and look ten years younger will proudly tell their age — but unless they're thin, most will never mention the numbers on the scale. Fit and fabulous tennis champion Serena Williams said in an interview that even she doesn't weigh herself because "it is too depressing."

A Citibank commercial illustrates how tongue-tied we become when faced with the issue of being overweight. In the advertisement, two heavy-set black women meet in the produce department at the supermarket. They haven't seen each other in some time. Sister A looks at Sister B's protruding belly and says something like, "When are you due?" Sister B looks like she is about to cuss out her friend. After a few embarrassing seconds she smiles and recites the Citibank slogan: "Thank you." The two women laugh and go about their business. The message is clear: Friendship is more important than any mention of weight that will cause hurt feelings.

"I don't talk to anybody about being fat," says Elizabeth. "I just try to handle it on my own." Denial and avoidance of communicating about our health issues are part of what keeps us trapped in shame and poor health. Because we as black women are used to being criticized, we put up our guard when people talk about ways we should improve. However, once we acknowledge the problem to ourselves we can heal our bodies and uplift our spirits. As they say in Overeaters Anonymous (OA), we are only as sick as our secrets.

Ebony OA

In 1998, as a long-time member of Overeaters Anonymous (see Chapter Eight), Octavia (not her real name) and her friends introduced "Ebony Overeaters Anonymous," an offshoot of the twelve-step fellowship specifically designed to address the cultural differences African Americans and Hispanics face as minorities who suffer from food addiction.

"I believe internalized racism is at the core of the compulsive overeating in the black community," says Octavia, who has a degree in black studies and has been a member of OA for over ten years. She recalls how childhood fears of racism led her to find comfort in food.

Growing up during the civil rights movement, she distinctly remembers when the little girls were blown up in the church in Birmingham, Alabama. "That really traumatized me," she says. "I became aware of racial issues and that some people hated me because of my skin color. It was a paradox for me. I grew up in a good Christian home and thought my character would be emanating from within. I asked myself, how could anyone possibly hate me without knowing me? I very much internalized the sense that I was different.

"I remember my family took a trip to Disneyland in Anaheim, which at the time was just about all white," Octavia continues. "I told my father, 'If we go to Disneyland, they are all going to stare at us.' I thought my family would be viewed as monstrosities . . . I literally had a mental breakdown. So we went across the street to Oscar's Big Boy hamburger stand and I had a burger and corn chips. I did what a lot of black people do. Rather than deal with the depression we may feel because of how we are treated in society, I learned to use food as a coping mechanism. . . . We don't know how to talk about [racism], or to either rage or take constructive action. Just as abuse of drugs and alcohol keeps us suppressed, so too does overeating. They are the modern chains of slavery, and when we misuse food and alcohol to cope, the white oppressors win."

Members of Ebony OA believe overeating is the way black people keep themselves "sated," and is another form of immediate gratification. "It's like when you know your taxes are due, but you just shove them in the drawer because you don't want to deal with them," Octavia explains. "We in the black community do the same thing with our problems. We use overeating as a way of denying and avoiding asking and answering the questions that are burning in our hearts: Am I really inferior? Do I really deserve to be hated because I am black?"

Octavia believes that by practicing the principles of Overeaters Anonymous — including admitting she is powerless over food — she has been able to get healthy by "learning to be black and stop trying to be white." Some people scoff at the notion of an addiction to food, but research has conclusively shown that both sugar and certain starches have addictive qualities. "When you never taste the food, but you just put it in your mouth because you feel compelled to eat, that's obsessive-compulsive behavior," she says. "If you eat and are never satisfied especially when you are not physically hungry, you may have psychological over-dependence on food."

Despite the fact that she is currently at her ideal weight and has maintained her weight loss for over a decade, Octavia realizes she is still addicted to food and remains heavily involved in OA. "I know firsthand the power of addiction. I remember eating honey-sweetened cookies, really healthy, right? Well not if you eat the entire bag and never taste them. Just being satisfied with my jaw moving up and down without ever really tasting the food was my way of stuffing my real fears and quieting nagging questions. Do I really have an IQ over 100? Is the Bell curve really true?"

As Octavia knows, admitting to out-of-control eating in the same way that alcoholics admit to the obsessive-compulsive nature of their drinking is not easy. However, in the forty-five years since OA began, thousands of overweight and obese people have found renewed physical health and have lost weight utilizing the concept of abstinence that is the basis of the program's recovery.[4] "Overeaters Anonymous offers a safe middle ground between surgery and doing nothing," says Octavia. "The problem is as a member of OA, it could take years to realize weight loss. We live in a get-it-done-yesterday world, and few want to go through the work of changing behavior and being patient. The fellowship will 'work if you work it.'"

The spiritual nature of all twelve-step programs means

depending on a Higher Power. Having been raised in the church, I know that the idea of trusting that God will handle things for us is easy and familiar for most black women. The hard part is that once we turn over our problems, we always think we know better and try to take them back, and do things our way. One definition of insanity is doing the same thing over and over again and expecting different results. "The spirit is willing but the flesh is weak" applies as much to our eating habits as it does to our intimate affairs. We can find the courage to make different choices and to see our world anew.

Ebony OA has both online and in-person meetings, a newsletter, and an annual retreat. Though OA has made great strides in reaching blacks and Latinos, progress is slow going because most decision-makers for the fellowship are white and not as cognizant of the special needs of minorities. Thus they resist changing the basic structure of the program, particularly the Eleventh Tradition, "The public relations policy is based on attraction rather than promotion." In other words, special outreach specifically to black and Hispanic communities is a no-no. However, because of the health concerns of minorities, groups like Ebony OA and various Spanish-speaking meetings are on the rise and still manage to stay within the broader traditions of the central groups.

I am a staunch believer in twelve-step fellowships and have personally witnessed many people released from the pain of addiction by working with a sponsor and regularly attending meetings where they share tears and fears, coping mechanisms, guilt, rage, doubt, and self-condemnation related to compulsive overeating. I am amazed at how a no-cost program comprised of volunteers can gather together for healing by religiously adhering to the precepts of "group conscience" and anonymity that are at the heart of all twelve-step programs.

With the prevalence of obesity in the black and Latino communities, it is time to make exceptional efforts to address these populations in ways that are culturally relevant. A one-size-fits-all approach cannot sufficiently address the obesity crisis. Blacks and Hispanics who struggle with their weight may not have access to quality medical care, may lack the ability to enroll in expensive gyms or eat special foods, or may struggle with a language barrier. Years ago, Bill W., the founder of Alcoholics Anonymous, went into the community and visited the homes of suffering alcoholics. He brought them good news that there is hope in sobriety. Ebony OA is extending this concept by going into the communities of populations that may not otherwise be aware of the benefits of OA. This approach should be lauded and encouraged. After all, isn't that what Bill W. once did?

Taking Stock

Addressing the reasons we are obese and at risk for weight-related diseases may mean taking an internal journey that is both scary and painful. Realize, though, it takes as much strength to suffer in silence as it does to open our minds and reach out for help:

- Clinical depression affects black women in great numbers,

but often goes undiagnosed and untreated. Depression can lead to distorted behavior, including compulsive overeating. If you believe you are clinically depressed, it is crucial that you get long-term counseling.

- Internalized racism may lead black women to use food as an escape. In order to achieve improved emotional, physical, and mental well-being, it's important that we honestly communicate our concerns to our families, to professionals trained to help us heal, and, most important, to ourselves.

- Obesity may be related to sexual problems, particularly if someone was sexually abused as a child. For those who use food as a way to cope with the pain of childhood sexual abuse, help is available.

- In trying to unravel and recover from the damage done by sexual abuse, the victim's family or significant other must also be involved in long-term counseling, so the whole family can heal.

Rob's Recommendations

No Secrets, No Lies: How Black Families Can Heal from Sexual Abuse, by Robin Stone, published by Harlem Moon, 2005.

Saving Our Last Nerve: The African American Woman's Path to Mental Health, by Marilyn Martin, published by Hilton Publishing, 2003.

Stolen Women: Reclaiming Our Sexuality, Taking Back Our Lives, by Gail Wyatt, published by Wiley, 1998.

Contrary to Love: Helping the Sexual Addict, by Patrick Carnes, published by Hazelden, 1994.

Black Rage, by William H. Grier and Price M. Cobbs, published by Bantam, 1968; reprinted by Wipf & Stock, 2000.

Courage to Change: One Day at a Time in Al-Anon II, published by Al-Anon Family Groups Headquarters, 1992.

Alcoholics Anonymous: The Big Book, Fourth Edition, by AA Services, 2001.

Hollywood's Finest

Woman Thou Art Loosed. Starring Kimberly Elise and Loretta Devine in the tragedy of an African American mother and daughter and sexual abuse in the family. 2004.

The Color Purple. Starring Oprah Winfrey and Whoopi Goldberg. Alice Walker's classic tale of abuse and redemption. 1985.

CHAPTER FIVE

Big Girls in La-La Land

Most plus-sized women are very aggressive and strong
because they have to struggle for most things. . . .
Size and color work against us.

—LORETTA DEVINE on achieving success as a
full-figured black actress in Hollywood

AS A KID, I watched Cathy cut up *Photoplay* magazine and
paste pictures of her favorite movie stars—Doris Day and Rock
Hudson—all over our bedroom walls. Movies, music, and celebrity worship had a profound effect on Cathy's life. I used to marvel
at how she knew all the words to a ton of musicals, like *Annie Get
Your Gun* and *West Side Story.* The ending of *To Sir With Love*
always brought a tear to her eyes, and she could not bear to miss a
bargain showing of *The Sound of Music* at the Rivoli Theater.

Cathy's favorite screen idol was another fifties bombshell,
Marilyn Monroe. Super-size portraits of the tragic blond god-
dess hung throughout Cathy's family home. Marilyn statuettes
were placed strategically on coffee tables; the famous painting

of Marilyn, James Dean, and Humphrey Bogart sitting at a lonesome café was displayed above Cathy's living room couch. No one knows quite where Cathy's Marilyn fascination came from; perhaps she identified with Marilyn's struggles with her weight and self-image and her misunderstood public persona. Or maybe, like Marilyn, Cathy had a sense her own body would not hold up long enough to see old age.

Cathy dreamed of being the next Diahann Carroll or a black Doris Day. But she settled for working in a number of plays and as a devoted stagehand behind the scenes at the Long Beach City College theater. I'll never forget when Cathy was in college and she practiced, until the wee hours of the morning, the haunting lines from Edgar Lee Masters's *Spoon River Anthology*, the tale of a Midwestern town whose residents speak to the audience from beyond the grave.

One passed in a fever,
One was burned in a mine,
One was killed in a brawl,
One died in a jail,
One fell from a bridge toiling for children and wife —
All, all are sleeping, sleeping, sleeping on the hill.

Black Earth Mother

The late, great Ethel Waters was a queen-size triple threat. Award-winning singer, actress, and writer, Waters, with her hallelujah smile and full figure, could make napkin-folding an act of dignity and determination. Outshining and outclassing the roles in which Hollywood cast her, Waters was at her best as the elegant, worldly-wise Bernice in the 1952 movie *The Member of the Wedding*. Playing the four-times-married housekeeper for a widower and his daughter, Waters defied the image of the servile, big black woman imprinted in American filmgoers' consciousness by Hattie McDaniel's character in *Gone with the Wind*. Thirteen years before *The Member of the Wedding*, McDaniel won the Oscar for Best Supporting Actress for her role as a slave serving the fussy Scarlett O'Hara.

Decked out in fox furs and cameo earrings in *The Member of the Wedding*, Waters redefined the image of African American women in Hollywood. Together with Dorothy Dandridge (the first black woman to be nominated for an Academy Award in the category of Best Actress for her leading role in *Carmen Jones* in 1954), Waters confirmed that black women could be as sophisticated and sassy as any of the lighter hued, skinnier, blonder women favored on the big screen at that time.

During the 1940s and 1950s with few exceptions, Hollywood treated big black women as the brunt of jokes or as old wise women and/or maids content to serve and revere white folks. The high-pitch-voiced Butterfly McQueen, best remembered for not knowing how to "birth no babies" in *Gone with the Wind*, also played Mammy with humor and defiance. Juanita Moore played a version of the wise nurturer/maid as the betrayed yet proud mother in *Imitation of Life*.

Waters, however, took the robust kindly caregiver character to another level in movies like *The Member of the Wedding*, *The Sound and the Fury*, and *Pinky*; her full-bodied insight and superior acting skills were too much for any stereotype to contain.

The Reliable Mammy

For years, big black women in the movies and on TV were usually presented as "mammies": characters who counseled, cooked, or chastised. An essay (published without author credit) entitled "The Cultural Image of the African American Woman" in the *Birmingham-Pittsburgh Traveler* describes that enduring image of fat black women this way:

> The Mammy was traditionally a large, dark African-
> American woman dressed in a calico dress with a bright
> do-rag on her head and a happy white smile on her face.
> She is submissive to her master or employer, but her outlets
> for aggressive behavior are African-American males, her
> mistress, and the white children of whom she takes care.[1]

In her book *Stolen Women,* Dr. Gail Wyatt writes that the mammy image endures because they are seen as "wise, asexual, non-threatening individuals whose values and desires, hopes and dreams were inseparable from those around her."[2] Wyatt, an expert on African American female sexuality, believes the mammy image is still visible today in the personas of "TV stars known for their friendly personalities and largesse" and cautions that "the mammy may have an unhealthy lifestyle of overeating. . . as a method of coping with the stress of poverty and the feeling of being unloved. . . ."[3]

While Cathy was too much of a risk-taker to be considered a mammy in the classic, negative sense, she may have internalized that characterization to some extent. She spent the last fifteen years of her life trying to make a difficult marriage work and struggling in the role of childcare provider for mostly white kids. Her spur-of-the-moment get-togethers and reputation for showering gifts on family members and friends were also well known. When asked to describe a favorite keepsake that Cathy had given, her close friend Bobbie exclaimed, "Everything in my house!"

Foxy Brown to Viveca Fox

Cinematic images of black women began to evolve as the film industry grew. During the height of the black power movement in the 1960s, audiences were introduced to a limber, physically fit shot-caller who served no one except herself. Pam Grier's larger-than-life portrayals in *Foxy Brown* and *Coffey* oozed a dangerous sex appeal and created black feminine vigilantism unseen before on the silver screen. Perhaps as a reaction to Grier's take-no-prisoners, gun-toting style, moviegoers in the 1970s fell in love with a lithe, sensitive, and vulnerable black woman in the accessible Diana Ross. The singer-turned-actress shone in her two most memorable roles: a skinny version of the musical genius Billie Holiday in *Lady Sings the Blues* and the love-over-career-choosing *Mahogany* ("success is nothing without someone to share it with") with costar Billy D. Williams.

In the late 1980s and early '90s, the explosion of marketing music via videos allowed black female entertainers like Janet Jackson, Little Kim, TLC, and Foxy Brown to declare their sexual independence with hard bodies and salty lyrics.

The late '90s and the new millennium brought a new crop of black actresses such as Sanaa Lathan (*Love and Basketball*), Queen Latifah, Jada Pinkett, Kimberly Elise and Vivica Fox (*Set It Off*), Vanessa Williams (*Soul Food*), Nia Long (*Boiler Room*), Regina King (*Jerry Maguire* and *Ray*). These women brought to life intelligent characters who were sexy in their complexity, in stark contrast to the one-dimensional mammy stereotypes.

Talking Fat in the City

The celluloid view of how African American women should act and what we should look like seeps into the consciousness of even the most outwardly confident sister. The power of the silver screen is so pervasive, it's no wonder that talk of dieting, exercising, and weight loss inevitably finds its way into any conversation in L.A. Women living in cities like Buffalo, Minneapolis, or Tempe shake their heads at Southern California's preoccupation with dieting. Tourists gasp at the idea of paying thousands of dollars to cut and sculpt new stomachs and cheeks, surgically erase laugh lines, pump up sagging rear ends, remove excess body fat, and staple stomachs.

Living in L.A. feels like being in a nonstop infomercial. Folks of all ages and hues buy or sell fitness and eternal youth. I can't count the number of my students who are models, personal trainers, actresses, future entertainment lawyers, up-and-coming hip-hop artists and producers, choreographers-in-training. To compete in show biz means looking the part: thin and buff. And catering to that image is big business. Sometimes it seems like everyone north of Wilshire Boulevard has a website and a plan for the next big thing to keep us forever young and thin. The HOLLYWOOD landmark sign perched high above L.A. is a promise and a warning, a way of life and a state of mind. Hollywood and its East Coast cousin, Madison Avenue, promote the perceptions of perfect people, places, and products. What they say is "hot," we, the public, buy.

So star-struck are Los Angelinos that even the police here aspire to look like actors, as do newscasters, gynecologists, root canal specialists, real estate agents, stay-at-home moms, waiters, gang members, and fallen priests. In the land of make-believe, you can be as bad as you wanna be, as long as you look good. Famous faces are everywhere; huge billboards of the hottest starlets rise high above Hollywood Boulevard, and star sightings in the Beverly Center or at a Lakers' game are as common as nonfat lattes. Gossiping about movie stars and aspiring to look just like them are two of the favorite pastimes of many people who live on the fringes of show business.

Living within a stone's throw of the sand, surf, and endless sun means wearing fewer clothes, a look that demands tightly toned flesh and hard bodies. High-paying jobs in the entertainment and high-tech industries and a mate who resembles your favorite star are as sought after as an orchestra-section seat at the Oscars.

Super Glo

In the 1992 movie A *League of Their Own*, a story about an all-female baseball league, the team manager (played by Tom Hanks) insists that there is "no crying in baseball." If criers are banned from baseball, the entertainment industry corollary would be "there's no fat in Hollywood." Fat and the silver screen do not mix. And plus-size black women behind the scenes in Hollywood are truly invisible women. With the relentless barrage of images of women who look nothing like those in most black families, it's no wonder young African American women are increasingly dissatisfied with their looks and lives. This discontent creates a yearning to look like the Hollywood dream factory's ideal of someone who is attractive, rich, and successful.

Hollywood rarely if ever reflects real life. However, *Waiting to Exhale*, based on the best-selling novel by Terry McMillan, created the kind of movie magic that had large black women around the world smiling and high-fiving.

The most memorable scene in the 1995 film occurs when Glo Matthews (played by actress Loretta Devine), having coyly chatted up her hunky neighbor, Marvin King (played by the late Gregory Hines at his finest), turns on her heels and struts away. The camera follows Glo for a few steps then pans in on Marvin, hypnotized by Glo's full swaying hips, his lips moist with anticipation. Feeling her suitor's gaze, Glo turns around and wriggles her fingers at Marvin in a playful, acknowledging wave.

"That movie validated me," says Jennifer, a statuesque African American aerospace worker, who was always self-conscious about her big behind until she saw Glo. (Jennifer also mentions the ode to big booties, Sir Mix-A-Lot's 1992 hip-hop tune, "Baby Got Back," as giving her the confidence to show off her rear end by wearing tight jeans.)

With *Waiting to Exhale*, Hollywood at long last depicts a big black woman as being sexy, desirable, intelligent, realistic, and confident. She has a sense of humor. But, unlike her counterparts in other films and media, Glo is not the butt of fat jokes. She is a full character, treated with respect. She even finds the happy ending — with Marvin, a good-looking, hard-working, supportive black man, the dream of so many black women.

Doing the Hollywood Shuffle

The first time Sheila ever wanted to write a letter to complain about a television show was when the caustic judge Simon Crowell of *American Idol* gave performers on the show a tongue-lashing and dismissed them for being too fat. In Sheila's view, the sisters were "thick but not obese. . . . He said nothing about how they sounded, just that they were too fat." Sheila realizes that Simon says what many people in Hollywood (and elsewhere) think and don't say: "Being fat is like committing a crime."

Sheila knows. An actor, producer, and agent in Hollywood, she is close to lining up the investors she needs for her first major production. Being a big woman working behind the scenes in Hollywood creates challenges for Sheila she's certain she would not face if she "looked like Halle Berry." Sheila goes on to say, "Since I look more like Star Jones, people see me and think I remind them of a cousin or an auntie, this jolly, happy person they would want to befriend."

Sheila says she considered weight-loss surgery, but rejected the notion, because she believes losing weight is "a mental thing, and that once I conquer that mental thing, I will be all right." Sheila believes her weight problems will be solved when she "retrains how I eat." Sheila's goal is to eventually "eat six small meals during the day, so I am not starving when I get home." Married with two children, Sheila says because of her hectic, stressful schedule she goes all day without eating and then winds up eating at "eleven or twelve at night."

Sheila knows that as a big black woman she has to take extra care with her appearance when she is taking meetings with all those "skinny stick figures" in Hollywood. She makes sure her suits are pressed and extra crisp, and her hair and makeup are "on tight." Sheila recognizes she must go above and beyond what a thinner person would do in order to counter the belief people have that overweight people are "automatically sloppy."

Recently, Sheila evaluated a script written by a young plus-size black woman who works for a well-known talk show host. The writer has been "a big girl all her life," Sheila says. The semi-autobiographical story is about the life and times of a talented black woman who happens to be big and trying to make it in Hollywood. In addition to the prejudices she confronts on the professional front, size also affects her personal life. On the verge of becoming a star, her boyfriend is instructed to "lose the fat girl." He does. Although potential movie investors "have shown heavy resistance to the concept," Sheila believes it will sell.

Angie and D'Angelo

The "lose the fat girl" script brings to mind the true-life saga of neo-soul singer D'Angelo and Angie Stone, the rhythm and blues vocalist who used to be D'Angelo's main squeeze. D'Angelo raised the pulse of millions of teen girls in 2000 when he appeared nude from the waist up in a video for his song called "Untitled." With heavy rotation on MTV and BET, the video showcased close-ups of D'Angelo's pulsing abs and rippling, muscular chest and biceps, along with his Prince-like screech. The video catapulted him from a successful balladeer into a best-selling artist and Grammy-winning icon.

Then the public learned that D'Angelo and Stone, with her silky chocolate skin, thousand-watt smile, and full figure, were a couple. D'Angelo's female fans started "hating on" Angie, who became the target of insults and slurs from Internet message boards to the dance clubs where couples cha-cha'd to D'Angelo's sensuous beat. Neither men nor women could imagine how the black Adonis could possibly be attracted to someone with a figure like Angie's. The singing couple just did not match the *EBONY* or *JET* fantasy of an equally yoked, beautiful black pair. Fans believed D'Angelo should be hooked up with a thinner and lighter-skinned woman than Angie Stone — or better yet, he should be totally single, available to fuel the fantasies of his panting female fans.

"It would be different if Angie looked like Jada Pinkett," one D'Angelo fan lamented. The haters went ballistic when they discovered that not only were D'Angelo and Stone involved in a three-year relationship but the couple also had a son together. Rumors swirled that Virgin Records had ordered D'Angelo and Stone to hide their relationship from the masses.

The pair eventually broke up. Some hardcore D'Angelo fans believe the split was caused by the music industry's need to portray D'Angelo as an eligible bachelor instead of what he was — a man in love with a woman who looks like many of his fans.

Despite the negative publicity, Stone's star kept rising. She went on to gain hundreds of thousands of loyal fans with her three albums, and in 2004 released *Mahogany Soul*, a CD on which she sang a duet with hip-hop luminary Snoop Dogg. (D'Angelo wound up in the tabloids in early 2005, looking dazed and bloated after being arrested for alleged drunk driving and drug possession.)

Neither D'Angelo nor Angie ever commented publicly about the details of their breakup. But the love affair of the plus-size singer and the buff crooner shows the power of image-makers in shaping tastes and turning celebrities into commodities.

Big Girls in Harmony

As women who are overweight know, there has always been a double standard when it comes to size. Even the words we use to describe a heavy man are less poisonous: "big boy," "husky," "stocky," and "rotund." Compare those to "cow" and "fat pig," and it's easy to see who's on the losing end. For women, size is often the first thing people notice and/or talk about.

Nowhere is the double standard more pronounced than in popular music. CD covers don't shy away from photographs of Christopher Wallace, also known as the Notorious B.I.G., a.k.a. Biggie Smalls (gunned down in L.A. in 1997), and his contemporaries "Big Pun" (who died of a heart attack allegedly due to his weight in 2000) and the best-selling rapper Fat Joe. Both

Notorious and Big Pun are legends in the hip-hop world and heavyset black men take no offense at being compared to them. Female fans swooned over Biggie Smalls and Big Pun the way they did over R&B superstar Luther Vandross at his heaviest. Size hasn't diminished the popularity of Ruben Stoddard, a heavyweight with a voice as smooth as butter, who a few years ago was voted an "American Idol" by millions of viewers of the popular TV show. No one ever mentions Barry White's girth while listening to his "baby-making" tunes that are favorites across generations.

Where are the female equivalents of Fat Joe or Luther Vandross or Barry White? Consumers of Billboard's hottest singles and music videos, along with global record conglomerates, don't seem ready to crown a heavy woman of any race as a pop princess. Those honors are reserved for thinner women like Grammy Award–winning R&B superstars Beyoncé, Alicia Keys, and *American Idol*'s Kelly Clarkson. Some would argue that full-figured vocalists like Jill Scott and Angie Stone have musical genius far beyond the talents of most women on today's Top 40 and should be fully promoted and appreciated as the multitalented artists they are. It's worth noting that legendary African American singers Bessie Smith, "Ma" Rainey, and Billie Holiday — large black women all — intoned from the depths of their spirit and birthed the blues, the art form that is the foundation of most of today's popular music styles. True soul knows no size, and thin should be no requirement for musical stardom.

Black Women Change the Channel

As African American women confront the obesity crisis in their private lives, show biz executives are wringing their hands over the changing television tastes of black women. TV viewership among black people in general and African American women in particular is in a free fall, according to a December 2004 report in *Mediaweek*, the bible of media and advertising trends. The audience for some shows, once popular with this demographic, has fallen as much as 68 percent. Even UPN (nicknamed the "united place for Negroes"), featuring such sitcom hits as *Girlfriends* and *All of Us*, has seen a steep decline in its African American audience.

The formula for television's bottom-line success is basic: Ratings determine advertising rates. A drop in ratings (i.e., fewer viewers) means fewer advertising dollars and less profit. When black viewers change the channel, network and cable programming goes into a tailspin.

Further describing how the big three networks (ABC, NBC, and CBS) have been affected by a slip in viewership among black females, *Mediaweek* cited the ABC sitcom *My Wife and Kids*, which was a hit with black audiences when it debuted in 2002. It is down a whopping 67 percent among black women ages eighteen to thirty-four. In addition, the trio of networks has shown "double-digit" declines among female soap opera viewers due in part to the 6 percent drop-off among black women in the demographic group most coveted by advertisers: ages eighteen to forty-nine.

[T]he problem is not confined to the broadcast networks.
BET (Black Entertainment Television), which is also owned
by UPN parent Viacom, is showing hefty season-to-date
ratings declines. BET is down 14 percent in total viewers,
down 25 percent in adults 18–34 ratings, 20 percent among
women 18–34 and 25 percent among women 18–49.[4]

Mediaweek quoted one worried TV honcho: "Something is
going on among African American viewers . . . and all networks
are being impacted in some regard, but there is no clear pattern.
We're baffled."

Oprah Winfrey is one of the most powerful women on and
off television, and the phenomenal success of her show has kept
her consistently atop the ratings. Although there could never be
another Oprah, eventually network executives may figure out
why black women are fleeing both daytime and prime-time TV
as viewers: because the sitcom world has worn out its welcome.
Upwardly mobile African Americans do not see themselves or
issues central to their lives reflected realistically. They are rejecting lame punch lines and tired stereotypes the way they would
a bad blind date. If network executives surveyed their program
offerings, they would find few black women starring in prime-
time roles, the notable exception being S. Epatha Merkerson of
Law & Order.

Even shows in the 1960s, '70s, '80s, and '90s portrayed black
women more positively. Who can forget Nichelle Nichols as

Lieutenant Uhura, the proud and sexy intergalactic navigator on the original *Star Trek?*

Where's the contemporary counterpart to Isabel Sanford's Weezy Jefferson, the wife of well-to-do entrepreneur George on *The Jeffersons.* Instead of playing a housekeeper, Weezie employed a maid, by the name of Florence, a role played with comedy and caring by Marla Gibbs, who went on to star in 227, a series that celebrated the importance of friends and family.

Shapely and ambitious Denise Nicholas played Council-woman Harriet DeLong on *In the Heat of the Night. The Cosby Show* and its spin-off, *A Different World,* featured black women as capable and successful professionals.

In *Living Single,* one of the most popular black sitcoms of the 1990s, Queen Latifah, Kim Coles, Kim Fields, and Erika Alexander were a foursome of friends who tackled real-life issues like racism and the corporate glass ceiling.

Predictably, the mammy image was well represented on TV through those decades too. The late Nell Carter's starring role in the '80s sitcom, *Gimme a Break!* featured the actress in the role of the black surrogate mother and housekeeper of the Kanisky family. The family consisted of the chief-of-police father, his three daughters, and later on a young nephew. For six years, Carter dispensed sage advice to all the Kaniskys while only occasionally revealing that she too had a family and a (love) life of her own.

America's celestial hope, Della Reese, star of *Touched by an Angel* in the '90s, brought a new twist to the maternal black woman characterization in her role as Tess. The heavyset cherub

Tess was "sent to earth to tell depressed and troubled people that God loves them and God hasn't forgotten them."

As television executives and programmers scramble to recapture the once-reliable black female audience, they might find a message in the increasing numbers of black women watching shows like *Star Trek: Enterprise* with its lone black male star, its emphasis on futurism, special effects, and a storyline that pits "species against species." Once an obsession of young white men, *Star Trek* has become a sci-fi favorite among African American women.

Could it be black women are hungry for more compelling, imaginative dramas instead of retread comedies and whitewashed reality TV? As Kevin Costner's character says in *Field of Dreams*: If you build it, they will come. Black women want television that provides ideas, concepts, and characters we can relate to, females who are big, bold, and brainy.

The Biggest Losers

Big black women need not apply when it comes to reality TV. Shows like *The Apprentice* and *Survivor* usually select slender black women with light skin. However, one niche in the reality genre, weight-loss TV, features large black women. *The Biggest Loser* and *Celebrity Fit Club* showcase large black women in their quest to shed extra pounds. Unfortunately, being featured on these shows feeds into the stereotype that all black women are fat and out of shape.

The Amazing Race reality show starred two super athletic

and physically fit African American couples that outlasted the competition and won a million dollars each. Unfortunately, their achievements came and went with little fanfare.

The question remains: How much reality is there on television when 65 percent of the American population is overweight but rarely represented on TV? And how much reality is there for black women, limited with few exceptions to weight-loss reality follies and token roles in the background?

The Mo'Nique Effect

One full-figured black star who represents a positive image for black women on television is actress and comedian Mo'Nique. Star of the UPN hit and *Moesha* spin-off *The Parkers*, Mo'Nique plays the flamboyant single mother of actress Countess Vaughn. The Parkers don't live in the 'hood as is typical of black TV families. They reside in the west side of L.A., and mother and daughter are classmates at Santa Monica Junior College.

Mo'Nique's success on *The Parkers* and *It's Showtime at the Apollo*, as well as in silver screen comedies *The Queens of Comedy* and *Soul Plane*, has earned her millions of fans. With these movies and her 2005 reality show *Fat Chance*, she has carefully cultivated an image of being big and loving. In her best-selling book, *Skinny Women Are Evil*, Mo'Nique writes about accepting herself as fat, even in Hollywood, where being small means being popular and getting paid big bucks:

What I've enjoyed is a lifelong love affair with every roll,
every lump, and every curve. And because I love me,
I've never felt the need to apologize for being my BIG,
BEAUTIFUL self.[5]

When young women of all races are asked to name a woman
who positively represents a big woman, they mention Mo'Nique,
along with Academy Award–nominated singer/actress Queen
Latifah, and, of course, Oprah.

Despite Mo'Nique's overall positive persona, some of the running gags on *The Parkers* are troubling and bring to mind tired
stereotypes of big black women. Mo'Nique relentlessly pursues
Stanley Oglevee, a nerdy professor, who "just wants to be friends."
He mocks and insults Mo'Nique's character every chance he gets.

Although Mo'Nique was quoted in an interview saying that
in real life she "could have the Professor anytime she wanted
him," the sight of her chasing the straight-laced bachelor, devising outrageous plots to win his affection, and dealing with his
put-downs feeds into the idea of the hard-up fat black woman
desperate for love.

The NAACP has awarded Mo'Nique the prestigious Image
Awards four times. Her on-screen and behind-the-scenes message
of self-love and ambition outshines formulaic sitcom scripts and
inspires black women hungry for positive role models.

Morning, Aunt Jemima

When it comes to product marketing, the large black woman has always been a popular selling tool. Perhaps the most famous presentation is the woman whose image has been a regular part of breakfast for more than a century. Aunt Jemima, with perfect white teeth and trusting eyes beaming from the front of millions of boxes of pancake mix and bottles of syrups, has gone places real-life black folks could never go. From the deepest reaches of the South to the toniest addresses on the west side of L.A., everyone loves Aunt Jemima.

Aunt Jemima's portrait has been updated over the years. That has not affected her popularity or that of her products. She has morphed from a bubble-cheeked mammy in a do-rag to a straight-haired, slender, and rouge-cheeked black career woman.

Using black characters like Aunt Jemima (and Uncle Ben) to sell foods has been a winning strategy for companies for years. Even today, who could ever associate Aunt Jemima the friendly black woman at the American breakfast table with diabetes, hypertension, and heart disease? Aunt Jemima is welcome in American homes, even while her real-life counterpart is invisible, typecast, and suffering poor health.

Rob's Recommendations

Skinny Women Are Evil: Notes of a Big Girl in a Small-Minded World, by Mo'Nique and Sherri A. McGee, published by Atria Books, 2003.

Naughty or Nice, by Eric Jerome Dickey, published by Dutton, 2003. A novel about the three large and lovely McBroom sisters, their big-time drama, and their men problems.

All of Me: A Voluptuous Tale, by Venise Berry, published by Dutton, 2000; reissued by NAL Trade, 2001. This novel explores the complexities of body image, weight, and self-esteem in the life of African American TV news reporter Serpentine Williams.

Hollywood's Finest

Chicago. Academy Award–nominated performance by Queen Latifah as a prison guard with pipes. 2003.

Waiting to Exhale. A film with Loretta Devine, Whitney Houston, and Angela Bassett, based on a best-selling novel (published in 1992) by Terry McMillan. 1995.

The Member of the Wedding. With Ethel Waters and Julie Harris. 1952.

CHAPTER SIX

Keeping Secrets, Taking Risks

Once you accept the fact that you're not perfect,
then you develop some confidence.
—Former First Lady ROSALYNN CARTER

TO THE REST of the world, it may have looked like Cathy's weight-loss surgery was a quick fix. But I don't think it was. From the moment she found out about the gastric bypass procedure, she saw it as a done deal, the end of years of torment about her weight.

Cathy's friends and relatives recall the euphoria she felt in the days leading up to the surgery, an elation that may have blinded her to the risks. They recall her frantic search for an insurance company to cover her operation, and her nose-diving spirits each time her application for coverage was rejected. She was turned down by at least three companies before one finally agreed to insure her and cover the operation.

Less than two weeks from the time she got insurance company approval, she was in the operating room. "I asked her specifically what kind of tests they gave her," recalls our sister Theresa, "and all Cathy said was, 'They made me get on a treadmill.' I don't believe she met the doctor that did the surgery more than once prior to going into the hospital."

"Cathy wanted the surgery done fast and she was trying to keep the fact she was having the operation away from her family," says attorney Michael Lotta, who has a reputation for taking on tough malpractice cases and winning justice and substantial judgments for his mostly minority clients. Contrary to what Cathy's friends and family maintain, Lotta — who filed a successful legal action against Cathy's doctors — believes he understands Cathy's primary reason for her rush to surgery. "Her husband would probably not have agreed to it, had he known," says Lotta, who communicated with Luke extensively during the lawsuit.

The world of gastric bypass surgery is changing fast. One major difference is that doctors now are more inclined to take on the so-called borderline patients who ten years ago they might have turned down. Doctors now receive less in insurance reimbursements than they once did. "Surgeons have to make up what the insurance companies are not paying," says Lotta. "So what you see are more and more surgeons taking the risk with 'iffy' patients. They insulate themselves by hiring 'clearance' doctors who give them the rubber stamp. That's what doctors did in Cathy's case."

Lotta adds, "Cathy's excitement to have the surgery as soon

as possible may have rubbed off on her doctor, who instead of waiting, allowed the operation to proceed." He feels the doctor is at fault ultimately, despite Cathy's desperation to have the gastric bypass. "It was the doctor's job to say, 'Yes, you may want it done in two days, because that's the perfect time for your business and you've made arrangements.' But the surgeon should have told Cathy in no uncertain terms, 'You are a high-risk patient and I can't sign off on [the operation] at this time.'"

Made Up and Prayed Up

Though Linda B. never knew Cathy, she knows all about how she died. The fact that you can lose your life from gastric bypass surgery has not deterred Linda B.'s efforts to get it done yesterday. Inside her plus-size body beats a full-figured determination to live life as a slender woman. At forty-nine, the same age Cathy was when she had the surgery, Linda B. is unhappy with her job, her on-again/off-again relationship with her boyfriend, her life, and her weight.

Linda B. has spent almost a year searching for an insurance company that will cover the $30,000-plus operation she believes will make her anew. She has discovered that as the mortality rate for gastric bypass grows, so too does insurance companies' reluctance to take chances on obese people looking for a surefire fix.

"I have no willpower," Linda B. says. "I have tried Weight Watchers, wiring my teeth, hypnotism, the drinks, the pills,

Jenny Craig, Fen-Phen. I have even tried Medifast, the so-called medical fasting. I can stick to the stuff for about a month but then I get hungry. I've prayed up and my mind is made up to have this operation."

She surfs the Net for hours researching the facts, figures, and stories about weight-loss surgery. One comprehensive gastric bypass site (obesityhelp.com) lists gastric bypass surgeons, doctors' specific training in bariatric surgical techniques, the number of years they've been practicing medicine and their specialty, AMA membership, office hours, office locations (some operate from more than one site), and testimonials from happy and some not so happy gastric bypass survivors.

The Tuskegee Disaster

For many years, African Americans were leery of even going to the doctor. Horror stories like the experiment on black men known as the "Tuskegee project" fueled skepticism of the medical profession, fears that have been passed down from one generation to the next. The 1997 film *Miss Evers' Boys*, starring Alfre Woodard, is based on the true and horrific story of the 1932 federal government study of syphilis and race. In Macon County, Alabama, 412 black men suffering from the disease were observed but denied any treatment in a misguided attempt to discover if black men reacted to the disease differently from whites. The men, "Miss Evers' Boys," unknowingly participated, and many suffered physical and mental breakdowns and eventually died excruciating deaths.

Eunice Evers was the African American nurse who cared for the men in the study. She took part in the duplicity by fooling her patients into believing the medicine they were receiving would cure them. Evers believed she was serving a "greater good" by proving to the world there was no difference in the way black men suffer.

The Tuskegee experiments have had a lasting effect in the black community. As recently as 2004, more than half of African Americans believed HIV/AIDS is a man-made virus created by the government to destroy blacks, according to research released by the RAND Corporation. The study found that many blacks are convinced that authorities are withholding a cure for the disease.[1]

The level of mistrust of the government among some African Americans is matched only by our suspicion of the medical establishment. But as African Americans move further from the Tuskegee nightmare and into the suburban middle class, and as more blacks enter the medical field, attitudes toward doctors are beginning to change.

Not long ago, most church-going folks lived by the adage, "If God meant for you to have a flat stomach, He would have given you one." Today, some young black women live by another adage when it comes to surgical improvements: "God helps those who help themselves."

Medical Disparities

For many African Americans and Latinos the idea of cosmetic surgery is totally out of the realm of our everyday existence, as we continue to struggle just to receive the most basic medical care. Statistics point out that African Americans in the inner cities receive their primary care in hospital emergency rooms and trauma centers.[2]

Twice as many working African Americans as working whites have no medical insurance.[3]

The disparity in medical care between blacks and whites extends well beyond the uninsured or underinsured. According to research published in 2004 in the *New England Journal of Medicine,* doctor training and inadequate attention to patients are two of the biggest factors affecting the quality of health care for African Americans and Hispanics. These factors contribute to higher mortality rates in minority communities.

Many African Americans with adequate insurance are poorly served by the medical community, according to attorney Michael Lotta. He has seen a sharp increase in the number of blacks and Hispanics seeking to file lawsuits for botched gastric bypass surgery. "I see every day that the quality of care for the African American is significantly less than the quality of care for the white population," Lotta says. "You will not generally see an affluent white woman come in with gastric bypass surgery complications. It has nothing to do with physiology. . . . It's because minorities receive inferior medical care overall."

By Any Means Necessary?

Sleep apnea, hypertension, and diabetes are a few of the so-called "comorbidities" insurance companies and doctors require diagnosis of in patients seeking gastric bypass operations. Weighing at least a hundred pounds over your ideal weight is another prerequisite. Stories abound of women who actually gain weight to reach the hundred-pound threshold to qualify for the operation. Linda B. watched one of her relatives pack on pounds to meet the minimum: "She was like eighty pounds overweight and she gained twenty pounds so that she could get approved for the surgery."

Sometimes people are rejected for the surgery because they weigh too much. Virginia, a mother of four, was using an oxygen tank to help her breathe because of her obesity; she also suffered from hypertension, congestive heart failure, diabetes, and sleep apnea. She was told she would have to lose weight to lower her blood pressure before she could have surgery, something she was able to do with relative ease.

"The doctors told me there were certain hospitals that wouldn't accept me because I weighed almost four hundred pounds," Virginia says. "My doctor said I had to lose forty pounds to bring my BMI into balance. I cried. If I could lose forty pounds, I would not be trying to have surgery. I went on a low-carbohydrate/high-protein diet and lost thirty-five pounds. Then I lost another thirty-five in the process of moving into a new home right before the surgery. I've lost eighty more pounds since the surgery . . . I still have a hundred pounds to go. The biggest change is that I don't have to sleep with oxygen anymore. I can move around and exercise. Before, I could not walk from the backyard to the front yard before I had to sit down and rest."

Although weight-loss surgery has become more acceptable, there is often a veil of secrecy about it. Some older folks in the black community still view "being cut" as vanity or as "trying to be white." The bias drives some people underground, not admitting to the procedure, and worse, not admitting to complications they suffer afterward.

Terri, a health-care worker from Houston, says she never considered surgery, but has "two friends who went through weight-loss surgery. . . . They are having problems now although they won't admit it."

Linda B. understands why women keep their decision to go under the knife hush-hush. "Most people will say, 'Oh God, please don't do this,' and women who want surgery don't want to hear that." Linda B.'s voice rises with passion as she declares, "You can tell me, 'Don't do it,' but I'm still going to do what I'm going to do. I just want to tell people beforehand, so in case something happens to me they will know what I went through."

Holding to the oft-quoted statistic of one death per two hundred gastric bypass patients, Linda B. believes the odds are in her favor. She is undaunted when she learns about the University of Washington study that puts the risk as high as one in fifty.

Linda B. still sees gastric bypass as her last, best resort to reach the weight of her dreams. For her and others, the decision to have the surgery becomes a metaphor for seizing control of their lives after years of being unable to manage their weight and feeling powerless to fight back when society punishes them for being fat.

In Stephanie's case, she says she never worried about being fat when she was growing up, despite her mother's relentless attempts to get her to diet. "I knew I would not be fat my whole life. I ate as much as I wanted. I knew I could fix it one way or another."

Some women who seek surgery undergo a phase similar to what psychologists call "addicted to the attraction phase" of a love affair. Like people at the beginning of a relationship when everything is candlelight and roses, they hear only what they want to hear. They spend hours dreaming of what their lives will be like as skinny people.

After Cathy died, friends looked at pictures taken of her right after the operation. Sitting up in her hospital bed, she wore a big smile, her hair in French braids, a hairstyle she never before wore. A new 'do for a new life.

Never underestimate the power of peer pressure. Most women having the surgery know friends or relatives who had it and lived to tell about it. Many also know of people who died as a result of the surgery, yet they forge ahead. Even two of Cathy's closest friends had gastric bypass operations within months of her death, gambling that tragedy would not strike twice within the same circle.

Most women who decide to have the operation have tried diets with the same vigor and single-mindedness. In fact, doctors and insurance companies require that potential patients document the weight-loss methods they've tried, such as Weight Watchers and Jenny Craig.

Facing the Music

After surgery, some women face a host of unexpected consequences, such as losing weight too slowly or too quickly, or losing and regaining weight. Women who experience dramatic weight loss often wind up distressed over the amount of excess skin hanging from their bodies.

Weight-loss surgery patients must also retrain themselves to eat slowly. Some have trouble adjusting to this and complain that food gets caught in their throat because they cannot chew and swallow the way they used to.

Depression and emotional letdown are other post-surgery realities, leaving some women with a feeling of buyer's remorse.

Thirty-nine-year-old Camille, a Los Angeles postal worker, said her prayers, gathered her nerves, and underwent an operation called a "modified gastric bypass," in which a "gastrostomy tube and a gastrostomy site marker" are placed inside her stomach.

At five feet four inches tall and 289 pounds, Camille yearned to realize her lifelong dream of being thin. "I always wanted to cross my legs," Camille laughs. She concedes that there are drawbacks to weight-loss surgery. A week after surgery, she had lost seventeen pounds and kept losing until she worried she'd "lost too much." A few months later, she still felt sick and depressed.

Camille says the doctors prepare patients for the physical aftermath of the surgery, but don't talk about the potential mental and emotional downside. Camille was especially upset over negative comments from co-workers when she returned to her job. She lost many "so-called friends" when she got thin. Camille has also found that now when she catches a cold, she "stays sick longer." Doctors are unsure why.

She mistakenly believes that since she's lost weight, there's no need to exercise. She is considering additional surgeries to remove the rolls of skin hanging from the back of her arms. "I still cannot wear sleeveless or even quarter sleeves," she says, a common complaint from women who have gastric bypass. Now a size 8 or 10, Camille says her arms are still nearly as big as they were when she weighed almost three hundred pounds.

In addition, Camille has to watch every bite she eats. Even though her stomach is cut to be smaller, she realizes it can and will expand if she overeats.

The Fine Print

Consider the complexity of gastric bypass: "The easiest way to describe the kind of gastric bypass surgery Cathy had is to imagine doctors taking two sections from your intestinal system," says attorney Lotta, "which is rather long, then cutting out a rather large segment of it and sewing it back together. Because of this, patients suffer a lot of post-operative complications, including infections, severe pain, swelling, and bowel obstructions."

With all the possible complications, you can imagine the amount of fine print that potential patients have to sift through. Prior to the operation, the potential risks are described verbally and on forms patients must sign. Doctors, insurance companies, and hospital personnel explain side effects and potential dangers in detail.

Some gastric bypass patients complain that the risks are downplayed during presentations from doctors and hospitals. Medical personnel involved in weight-loss surgery tend not to dwell on the negative side effects. It's up to patients to educate themselves thoroughly, be realistic, and ask questions.

Many women report that they ignore the fine print. All the medical and legal mumbo jumbo makes most people's eyes glaze over. Occasionally, women hear about the risks and reconsider. One twenty-year-old woman who had her surgery already scheduled had a last-minute change of heart and cancelled it after talking with someone who'd had the procedure. That patient broke down in tears, distraught over the speed at which she was losing weight.

Gastric bypass surgery can end in joy or in tragedy. Each woman must decide for herself if the potential benefits outweigh the risks. "I would not have that surgery on a cold day in hell," says Lotta, who has seen his share of gastric bypass disasters. "It's just too risky."

Not All Surgeons or Hospitals Are Created Equal

Cathy's surgeon is a prominent Beverly Hills physician. He continues to perform gastric bypass operations, despite Cathy's death, the lawsuit our family filed, and its settlement. According to Lotta, doctors who perform high-risk surgeries, such as gastric bypass, usually have other doctors sign off on the operation beforehand.

"What really caused Cathy's death was that the doctor who did the gastric bypass surgery, recognizing [Cathy] was a high-risk patient (all gastric bypass patients are basically high risk), obtained not one, but two surgical clearances, including one by a cardiologist," Lotta recalls. "The cardiologist recognized that Cathy had a heart problem that was not appropriately treated. Therefore she should never have cleared her for the procedure because it is an elective one." A necessary, nonelective procedure might have been considered a justifiable risk. However, elective procedures for a patient with a major untreated condition are usually rejected until the condition is addressed. The four-hour surgery taxed Cathy's heart.

In 2002, the *Fresno Bee*, an award-winning Central California newspaper, ran an excellent, thought-provoking series by reporter Tracy Correa on the risks of gastric bypass surgeries. One of the articles, entitled "Key Questions to Ask Before Having Bypass," suggests prospective patients "ask the surgeon how many of his patients have died or required corrective surgery. Be alert to a doctor who wants to quote national statistics instead of his own; a reputable doctor tracks his patients months and years following surgery."[4]

This is a reasonable precaution. However, few doctors will admit that any patients have died as a result of weight-loss surgery. Rather than querying the physician directly, you can contact your state board of health, which lists information concerning "infractions" and other penalties doctors receive. Bear in mind that even this kind of research can be incomplete. For instance, in California, if a doctor settles a case for less than $30,000, no official record is available. (Regulations and procedures for reporting medical infractions differ from state to state.)

As part of the *Bee* series, Correa also did exhaustive reporting on the three Fresno Valley hospitals in which thirteen patients died as a result of gastric bypass surgeries between 2000 and 2002. Dr. Alan H. Pierrot, founder of the Fresno Surgery Center, which was mentioned in Correa's story, took exception to the series' investigation into the lack of quality care in medical facilities. In a letter to the editor, Pierrot wrote:

> Both medical ethics and insurance underwriters require
> that patients be informed of the serious risks of surgery.
> Documenting informed consent is the first line of defense
> against a frivolous lawsuit. I will wager the cost of a full
> page ad that in the medical records of the patients *The Bee*
> identified as having bad outcomes, there is clear preoperative
> documentation that the patients were fully informed as to
> the possibility of the complications. . . .[5]

"Preoperative documentation" was part of Cathy's file. All the risks and dangers are usually spelled out, in a way similar to the litany of risks listed at the end of drug commercials on TV. And just as we do when we take our prescription drugs, we tempt fate and reason that bad things happen to other people. After all, who would agree to any surgery if in their heart of hearts they thought they would die on the operating table or from something as seemingly innocuous as an infection a few days later? But gastric bypass is high-stakes business, and people who are at least one hundred pounds overweight with a comorbidity are automatically at greater risk.

It's important to recognize there are many people, seen and unseen, involved in every kind of surgery — from the surgeon and anesthesiologist to the nurses and technicians who maintain the hospital equipment.

Correa suggests that when considering gastric bypass, a patient should "find out whether the hospital where your surgery will be performed has the equipment to identify post-surgery problems. For example, does the hospital have a CAT scan machine — a critical piece of equipment for detecting potentially deadly abdominal leaks?"[6]

There's a mountain of paperwork involved in any surgery. Just like signing documents to buy your first home, the devil is in the details. If there's a term you don't understand, ask the doctor to translate it into laywoman's language. Understand the fine print. Don't be embarrassed or feel foolish. Tour the hospital and ask to meet the nurses who will be involved in your aftercare. If you're not satisfied, walk away. Trust your gut feelings.

Virginia, the woman who once had to use oxygen, says that at first she was going to have the surgery in San Diego, but decided against it because her doctor told her it was too far from her home in Los Angeles County. "You're going to have complications and we'll have to rush you back," he warned. Other doctors Virginia contacted "just did not seem like they cared about me as a person too much." She finally settled on a doctor referred to her by the University of Southern California Medical Center. He ran a series of tests the other doctors did not, including sending her to a heart specialist. Virginia says he even referred her to an internist who did a colonoscopy.

If you feel like being extra bold, check out whether there is a malpractice attorney willing to consult with you about what typically goes wrong with weight-loss surgeries. Things might have turned off differently for Cathy if she had spoken to a reputable, experienced malpractice attorney like Mike Lotta before going ahead with the operation.

Malpractice Lawsuits

America has become known as a "sue-happy society." People who feel they have been wronged by hospitals and/or doctors believe the erring party should pay. Families of patients who die or are harmed by poor medical treatment often turn to the courts in hopes of finding justice and a lofty judgment to ease their suffering.

President George W. Bush began his second term in 2005 by vowing to halt so-called "junk lawsuits." He wants to see caps placed on damages awarded by a jury for malpractice pain and suffering, limiting them to $250,000, effectively ending multimillion-dollar awards. (The Bush proposal would allow unlimited damages to cover economic losses. In other words if something goes wrong with your operation, you [or your family] may only get damages to cover losses related to your earning potential. If you are unemployed or working at home taking care of your family, "economic losses" could be a lot less than your pain and suffering.)

L.A. Law

Just as all surgeons and medical centers are not equal, so too the scales of justice are often weighted against African Americans and other minorities. Because of his insight and expertise, Lotta settled the case against Cathy's surgeon and his "clearance" doctor quietly — albeit for six figures. Lotta, who is white, decided not to go to trial in Cathy's case because of the harsh realities he has learned during his fifteen years of malpractice litigation. "We live in a very corrupt legal system," Lotta states. "The wrongful death statute allows for one recovery for death and the maximum of $250,000 in general damages, that is the loss of the life. In Cathy's case, the other side [the doctors' attorneys] understands that they could get hit for $250,000, so they might find a doctor who will testify falsely for another doctor to help make their case for innocence.

"In my experience civil juries are generally not as sympathetic [to the complainant] as they once were," he says. "African Americans are not treated fairly. . . . Because of the demographics in Los Angeles County, many civil panels hearing malpractice lawsuits are predominately white. Jurors are human and some bring their racial prejudices and other biases to deliberations. Unfortunately, the attitude I've encountered, having interviewed thousands of potential jurors, is something akin to 'we aren't going to give that interracial couple, like Cathy and her husband, a lot of money,' because according to the bigots, 'we just killed another black person. Her life isn't important. We will side with the doctor.' It sounds terrible, but it's the reality of courtrooms."

The Bottom Line

Haste, denial, and ignorance can lead to potential disaster when undergoing such a major surgery as gastric bypass. Unfortunately, there's a disparity in the way black people are treated in the medical world as well as the courtroom. This may mean the odds of something going wrong could be greater for a black woman and she may have little legal recourse. Knowledge is power. The more you know, the better your chances are of being a survivor rather than a victim.

If you are overweight or obese and believe that the end justi-
fies any means, consider the following:

- *Different procedures for surgeries.* "Some surgeries are so
  restrictive the patient has to be taught exactly what to eat, bit
  by bit," explains Dr. Mal Fobi. "Those are the simple surgeries. As you get into the more complicated surgeries, you have
  the 'feedback' systems, so that if a patient eats certain things,
  she literally gets sick. This stops her from eating and she loses
  weight. The more complicated surgeries have the feedback
  systems because the patients are less likely to comply (on
  their own). With these complex surgeries patients will comply, whether they want to or not, because if they eat certain
  foods they will get sick."

  The National Institute of Diabetes and Digestive and
  Kidney Diseases (NIDDK) of the National Institutes of
  Health, the federal government's lead agency responsible for
  biomedical research on nutrition and obesity, offers the following description of the process of bariatric surgery:

  These operations combine creation of small stomach pouches
  to restrict food intake and construction of bypasses of the
  duodenum (the first segment of the small intestine) and other
  sections of the small intestine to cause malabsorption. . . .
  This causes reduced calorie and nutrient absorption.[7]

  The "malabsorptive technique" of bariatric surgery that
  both Virginia and Cathy had is the most restrictive in terms

of the foods and nutrients that are absorbed into the body. It carries the highest risk of complications, according to the NIDDK.

The "adjustable gastric banding," also known as the "lap band," is a procedure in which a hollow band made of special material is placed around the upper end of the stomach; the band can be tightened or loosened over time to change the size of the passage.

"Vertical banded gastroplasty," so-called "stomach stapling," utilizes both a band and staples to create a small stomach pouch.

The "laparoscopy" technique is popular because it can be done quickly and causes less scarring, involving only one or more small incisions. However, even this less invasive procedure can be dangerous, according to Lotta. The surgery requires the doctor to look through a microscope an inch in diameter at the entire abdomen and intestinal system, which creates a higher risk for an untoward event. "There are lots of organs inside you that can be clipped during a laparoscopic operation," Lotta explains. "Something could get accidentally nicked — perhaps a gallbladder, or a kidney, or a uterus. These mistakes happen. They are not uncommon."

- *Keloids.* Raised scars or keloids are not exclusive to black people, but African Americans know all too well their pain and embarrassment. Technically known as hypertrophic scars, keloids occur from skin injuries such as surgical incisions, traumatic wounds, vaccination sites, burns, acne, or even minor scratches. Young women, African Americans, and other dark-skinned people are most susceptible to keloidosis, a condition in which multiple or repeated keloids are produced. Although keloids may flatten and become less noticeable over time, they can become irritated and/or large and disfiguring.

Some gastric bypass techniques require incisions from below the breasts to just beneath the naval. If you are prone to keloids, you may want to consider potential scarring when making your decision. While not life threatening, keloids can be distressing and unattractive.

- *Flabby to the bone.* Overall, Virginia was happy with the results of her surgery. She felt like she'd been spiritually and physically born again. However, there is one thing she wishes her doctors had explained more thoroughly beforehand. Because she has lost so much weight, Virginia must have additional surgeries to, in essence, reconstruct her whole body.

"I am going to have several more operations: a tummy tuck, breast reconstruction, an inner thigh and outer bilateral thigh operation, in addition to surgery to remove flab around my hips and butt," she says. "Unfortunately I got really bad keloids from the surgery and since I have to have my breasts done, I am researching a new technique for breast reduction, no stitches or staples. Medicare will pay for the breast surgery and the tummy tuck. The bilateral hip and thigh operation, I will have to pay for. So far, Medicare and my back-up insurance coverage have paid for all of the nearly $200,000 cost of the surgery and aftercare. But I will have to pay thousands more for the reconstructive operations I need."

Virginia describes her skin as loose and wrinkly, a consequence she never heard mentioned at seminars she attended before the surgery. As a big fan of the *Extreme Makeover* TV show, Virginia wondered if this might be a side effect. "People say all you have to do is exercise," she says, "but once you reach a certain age, that skin is not coming back to elasticity. It's going to wrinkle, sag, and hang. The downside is when I look at myself naked — it's like a horror story. Of course, when you see yourself naked at four hundred pounds, that's no pretty sight either. I was hoping to get on a makeover reality show, tell my story, and get them to pay for all my additional surgeries."

- *Weight loss reversed.* Even having surgery doesn't guarantee permanent weight loss. "The surgery can be beaten," says Dr. Fobi. "Gastric bypass is supposed to work by allowing you to take five hundred to six hundred calories per meal. But you can eat a meal at six o'clock and then have a meal at seven, then have a meal at eight, and a meal at nine, ten, eleven, and so on. You can eat five six hundred–calorie meals, which add up to three thousand calories. Then you start all over. . . . So you can easily eat 7,500 calories even after having the surgery. For some, the surgery is there for them to beat.

   "We are hoping that people who sit down to eat breakfast," he continues, "will do what people who successfully keep the weight off do. For example, post-op, a woman will take three hundred calories for breakfast and feel full. By the time she is hungry again, it is lunchtime, so she eats three hundred more calories. And at dinnertime she will eat a meal worth three hundred calories and be full. By the end of the day she has eaten nine hundred calories, instead of six thousand. So the surgery is a tool to reinforce behavior modification."

Few of the many doctors performing these surgeries deny the potential for weight gain after surgery. Dr. Kevin Brown of the Crenshaw Health Expo says he regularly sees black women who have had gastric bypass and come to him because they have gained the weight back.

If someone is a chronic overeater before the surgery and doesn't change her eating habits afterward, she's bound to regain the weight. It's important to get to the root problem of why a person is obese in the first place, which is why pre- and post-surgery counseling are so crucial.

Debra, a forty-seven-year-old African American security guard and mother of four, battled her weight most of her life, just like Cathy had. She too was at her wit's end when she took a chance on weight-loss surgery. Debra recalls being a "lonely child" constantly teased and taunted because she was big. In the early 1980s Debra decided to undergo a new kind of operation that a friend told her could help her to slim down permanently. "I would never have that kind of surgery again," she says more than twenty years later. She regained nearly all of the one hundred pounds she lost within a few years after she had "stomach stapling."

Unfortunately for Debra, she was operated on at a time when the procedure was neither popular nor perfected. When she had it, she was in a bad relationship with her oldest child's father and her mother was dying. She became suicidal. After the surgery, Debra still had the same problems in her life, compounded by new, physical ones.

"I had to wear a diaper because, in some way, the surgery affected my bowels," she says. Although some gastric bypass patients need to have the surgery redone for one reason or another, Debra couldn't afford a second surgery. To this day, she still battles her weight and incontinence. Debra tells any woman who asks her to try Herbalife food supplements to lose weight instead of having a weight-loss operation.

- *Pregnancy.* Debra says when she got pregnant after her gastric bypass, she was afraid to eat because she was afraid she would undo her stomach staples. Because she ate so little, her baby didn't get the proper nutrition and was born prematurely. Most medical professionals, however, see Debra's case as an anomaly and report no direct connection between complications during pregnancy and gastric bypass. However, many doctors recommend women wait at least a year after surgery before becoming pregnant to give the woman time to stabilize her weight. One dietician from USC who works with bariatric patients says the surgery actually has a positive effect for women wanting to have children because many overweight women have problems with infertility or with carrying their baby to term, according to obesityhelp.com. If you are thinking about becoming pregnant before or after weight-loss surgery, be sure to talk to your doctor about the risks.

Rob's Recommendations

Livin' Large: African American Sisters Confront Obesity, by Stacy Ann Mitchell and Teri Mitchell, published by Hilton Publishing, 2004.

The Patient's Guide to Weight Loss Surgery: Everything You Need to Know About Gastric Bypass and Bariatric Surgery, by April Hochstrasser, published by Hatherleigh Press, 2004.

Am I Thin Enough Yet? The Cult of Thinness and the Commercialization of Identity, by Sharlene Hesse-Biber, published by Oxford University Press, 1989; reprinted in 1997.

Hollywood's Finest

Standing on My Sisters' Shoulders. A documentary about the commitment, passion, and perseverance of women in Mississippi during the civil rights movement. 2003.

CHAPTER SEVEN

Latinas: Our Bodies, Ourselves

How much does our body know that we know not?
Can it be cajoled to release its secrets?
—Chicana writer PAT MORA

IF THE NUMBER of Overeaters Anonymous (OA) programs sprouting up all over the globe is any indication, the problem of fat has spread far beyond America's borders. There are OA meetings in more than sixty countries, including African nations such as Nigeria and Kenya, and in places with so-called Afro Latino populations, like Panama, the Dominican Republic, Puerto Rico, and Costa Rica, where my mother was born. In Mexico alone, fifty meeting times are listed on the OA website. Weight Watchers International also holds meetings in Mexico, Brazil, and South Africa.

According to Dr. Fobi, black women around the world are suffering from obesity. "Once a populace becomes a bit elitist," he says, "they are going to have an ability to acquire food and store it rather than use it." While Africa usually brings to mind images of starvation and famine — Niger, Ethiopia, Zimbabwe, Zambia, Mozambique, Lesotho, and Swaziland are devastated by these conditions — there are places in Africa (for example, Nigeria and South Africa) where obesity is becoming a concern.

Globally, more than one billion people are now officially classified as overweight or obese, according to the World Health Organization (WHO). Fast food is a reality worldwide. At the beginning of the twenty-first century, McDonald's held a 63 percent market share of junk food sales in the 117 countries where it was located, approaching Coca-Cola in its international reach.[1]

With rapidly changing entertainment technology leading to less physical activity and an increased appetite for fast food, problems of obesity and weight-related diseases will grow. Many experts believe the fast food diet is the primary reason for the increase in obesity in the United States and overseas. As a result, WHO has taken steps to promote health education and awareness in developing countries.

In Panama, where many of my cousins still live, hypertension and diabetes, rather than obesity, are the major health issues, despite diets rich in homegrown papayas, mangos, watermelons, and bananas. Their meals also include a lot of fish reeled in fresh every day. But an overabundance of fried foods and lack of preventive health care result in diet-related diseases. My earliest memory of my Costa Rican grandmother is of her holding her chest and taking small white pills for her heart.

Women in Latin America who never worried much in the past about watching their weight are now increasingly troubled by high rates of hypertension, cancer, and heart disease, which can lead to early death. On the plus side, physical activity is very much interwoven into daily life in developing African nations and in countries like Costa Rica and Mexico. Round-trip hikes on foot from home to work, fewer cars and more bikes, children who play outside without fear of abduction, and a variety of strenuous household chores are part of the culture. However, just as in the United States, high-calorie foods increasingly contribute to poor health in Afro Latino families.

For example, fried pork, cow tongue, chorizo, refried beans, oil-drenched tortillas, cheesy burritos, and tamales are the staples of some Latino meals here and abroad. In cultures dominated by machismo, the desire to win male approval even has a seat at the family dinner table. One young Chicana says she was taught that as soon as the man of the house finishes eating, the woman should immediately remove his dish. That way he "does not have to look at a dirty plate."

Most women hearing about the rush to remove a dish would probably roll their eyes. However, many of those same traditions and ideas are alive and well in Latino cultures throughout the United States, affecting the way women treat themselves and view their bodies.

Latinos: The Majority Minority

The melting pot that is the United States grows increasingly diverse and less Eurocentric demographically. One need only look at the statistics to see the critical role Hispanics play in this shift. According to the U.S. Census Bureau, the U.S. Hispanic population has reached almost 40 million (nearly 14 percent of the total population), making it the nation's largest ethnic minority.

Sixty-seven percent of U.S. Hispanics are of Mexican heritage. Nearly a third of Hispanics, though, trace their ancestry to other nations. In fact, 10 percent identify ourselves as Afro Latino, having both Hispanic and African ancestry, a group becoming more and more recognizable. Popular Afro Latinos include baseball slugger Sammy Sosa, actress Rosie Perez, the late Cuban salsa singer Celia Cruz, and *The Fresh Prince of Bel-Air* star Tatyana Ali.

The increase in numbers of Hispanics in the United States is not only changing the American cultural landscape, it is also changing the way Hispanics look. Weight, both real and perceived, is an integral part of daily life.

The Gender Divide

Yasmin Davidds-Garrido is the author of the groundbreaking *Empowering Latinas: Breaking Boundaries, Freeing Lives*, a powerful firsthand account of her quest for self-determination and what it means to be Latina in patriarchal cultures. Davidds-Garrido believes weight and body image struggles begin early for most Latinas. Similar to African American women, Latinas with extra weight are viewed as mother figures. For black women and Latinas, serving delicious meals is a way to show love to friends and families. Their culinary prowess and caretaking skills make them the most important member of their families and help them feel content with their place in the world.

Yet Latinas, like other women, encounter contradictory messages — sometimes from the culture at large and sometimes in their own homes — leading young girls to believe "our bodies are one thing and our 'selves' are something completely different," says Davidds-Garrido. Whereas African Americans often speak of a matriarchal familial structure, in Latino cultures the man is boss — adored, feared, and revered. Thus, girls are constantly waging psychic and emotional war against what Davidds-Garrido calls "body image/sexuality" because young Latinas are taught they are born to be "sex machines" made for male pleasure and for bearing children. This reflects a basic disconnect in Latino culture that discourages women from feeling comfortable with their own physical being and makes them depend on men to determine their self-worth, says Davidds-Garrido, a counselor to young Latinos focusing on a wide range of topics including domestic violence and body image.

Experts believe that Latinas must unlearn their cultural conditioning that encourages them to sacrifice themselves to please men. Lessons learned in childhood come from watching mothers, aunts, and female friends work hard to earn a husband's or boy-friend's compliments about her delicious cooking, her house cleaning, or her child rearing. This male orientation makes it difficult for young girls to develop basic feelings of value beyond their role of serving men. Observing the female response and the way it is reflected in the need for male approval, a young woman comes to devote herself to pleasing men even at the expense of her own self-love and emotional well-being.

Davidds-Garrido's personal experience reflects the mixed messages between the traditional and individual ideals. Her father, who was from Ecuador, regularly weighed her on a scale when she was a child. "If I did not lose weight, he would beat me," Davidds-Garrido recalls. "Dad was overweight himself, and he would say to me, 'No one likes fat little girls.' So I grew up with the feeling that unless I was skinny, no one would love me."

She suffered from eating disorders as a teen, using "diet pills and every weight-loss program there is. My weight has been an issue my whole life. Only in the last few years have I come to terms with my body and really embraced it — especially now that big behinds like J.Lo's are in; that has really helped."

Carmen, a social worker in Orange County, California, was born in the Dominican Republic. In 2003, she underwent gastric bypass surgery. She recalls her eating habits being scrutinized by an overbearing parent while she was growing up. Weighing ninety-five pounds at age sixteen, Carmen says she was a "picky eater," and remembers her mother's attempts to fatten her up: "My mother would sit next to me with a belt. I had to eat everything on my plate, plus a glass of milk. Only then would she stop bugging me. In Latino culture they pretty much force food on you." Carmen's weight ballooned due to a combination of fatty, fried food and lack of exercise.

Natalie earned a PhD from the University of Southern California and currently runs a senior citizen nutrition program in Los Angeles. She has mixed memories about growing up fat in a Mexican American household. Through OA, she came to grips with the pain of her childhood and has lost one hundred pounds, weight loss she has maintained for more than ten years.

Immigrating from Mexico, Natalie's father was a farm worker and her mother worked as a seamstress in Los Angeles to support their family of seven. Theirs was the rough road many Mexican American immigrants travel pursuing the American dream. With both parents working long, hard jobs, eldest children, like Natalie, are given responsibility for taking care of younger siblings. Food became Natalie's way of burying her feelings of being overwhelmed by the adult responsibilities that were a part of her daily life.

"I'm in my forties, now," she says, "so I'm not sure how it is for the current generation of young people. But when I was growing up, children were seen and not heard. I had uncles who were alcoholics, and I watched their wives suffer severe domestic violence because of it. Most of the women coped either as 'martyrs' or by eating their way out of their misery.

"You're raised traditionally celebrating everything with food; at the same time when you start to gain weight, you feel ashamed," she continues. "Relatives say, 'Gee, you're such a pretty little girl, but you're letting yourself get so fat,' at the same time they're

LATINAS: OUR BODIES, OURSELVES

feeding you more and more. When my aunties saw that I became distorted in terms of body size, I heard them talk about me. . . . It was painful. There wasn't any support or anyone saying, 'You're a beautiful little girl, we are here to help you.'"

At school, she remembers wanting to fit in. Like many of her classmates, she wanted to join the Girl Scouts. "I asked my mother if I could join," Natalie recalls. "I wanted to do something like everybody else. She said, 'We don't join Girl Scouts . . . you know you have brothers and sisters. You don't need that.' I felt a definite level of disconnection with my peers and that disconnect was exacerbated by the fact that I was becoming an obese teen. At five feet six, I weighed 240 pounds. Starved for any kind of attention, I got pregnant when I was sixteen."

When her daughter was seven years old, the child was shot, paralyzing her from the neck down. Natalie then heard something from doctors that changed her life in more ways than one. They told her, "You are responsible for this child, you are responsible for whether she lives or dies, by your care and the decisions you make about her care."

"No one had ever said to me I was truly responsible," Natalie says. "I was always real good at eating my way through things and suddenly food was no longer an option [for escape]. My daughter was not going to walk again and the choices I made would affect the rest of our lives.

"Now when I'm speaking to Latino women in small groups in East L.A. or even in various other capacities — especially when my daughter was young and I was dealing with a lot of parents with traumatically ill children — the majority are obese Hispanic women. I talk to them about taking care of their children, but I also tell them about how I used food to cope. Without judging them I explain what I had to do in order to be present for my daughter. Many of these women are in households where the husband is an alcoholic or a drug addict or abusive. Many married young and are quite innocent. Many have taken to food as if it were a pacifier. Their eating and their children give them reasons to live."

Natalie got divorced a year after her daughter's accident. During the course of her marriage, she never heard her husband make a comment about her weight, even though she often felt depressed about it. After the divorce, he commented to someone, "Yeah, she waddled," a remark that shamed her and continued to hurt even after she lost a lot of weight.

For the last fifteen years, Natalie has worked out every day and her size 6 body shows it. "I realize now that all the time I was obese I was still attractive, but I had so much shame about my obesity," she says. "Now that I'm small, I see the attention I get, especially from Hispanic males. It definitely affects the way they treat you. I've seen the wives of these men just kind of look away when the men eye other women, and my heart just bleeds for them."

Coming to America

Because many Hispanics have immigrated to the United States relatively recently, their patterns of obesity are more easily traced than those of African Americans and other groups. Not surprisingly, obesity among Latinas is a U.S. phenomenon.

A 2004 study by the Harvard Medical School revealed that obesity is relatively rare in foreign-born residents until they've lived here for a period of time:

> Only 8 percent of immigrants who had lived in the United
> States for less than a year were obese, but that jumped to
> 19 percent among those who had been here for at least 15
> years. That compared with 22 percent of U.S.-born residents
> surveyed . . . The link between obesity and numbers of years
> in the United States was found in white, Hispanic and Asian
> immigrant groups. It was not seen in foreign-born blacks,
> but their numbers in the study were too small to draw any
> conclusions.[2]

The effect of life in the U.S. on immigrants involves a complex set of factors — for example, our nation's car culture, a more sedentary lifestyle, fast food, highly processed, high-calorie foods, and everyday stress.

Also contributing to weight issues is the financial struggle some new immigrants experience. Studies have shown a definite correlation between poverty and obesity among both African Americans and Latinos. According to the American Obesity Association (AOA), low-income minorities appear to have the greatest likelihood of being overweight. The AOA reports the following:

- Among women, the black (non-Hispanic) population has the highest prevalence of overweight (78 percent) and obesity (50.8 percent).

- Among men, the Mexican American population has the highest prevalence of overweight (74.4 percent) and obesity (29.4 percent).

- The prevalence of overweight, obesity, and severe obesity (BMI of 40 or more) increased for men and women in various racial/ethnic groups in the U.S. over the last decade.

- Diabetes has been reported to occur at a rate of 16 to 26 percent in Hispanic Americans and black Americans, aged 45 to 74, compared with a rate of 12 percent in whites (non-Hispanic) of the same age.

- Among Mexican Americans, obesity and type 2 diabetes are both increasing, unlike other risk factors of cardiovascular disease, including smoking and high blood pressure, which are declining.

- Cultural factors related to dietary choices, physical activity, and acceptance of excess weight among African Americans and other racial/ethnic groups appear to play a role in interfering with weight-loss efforts.[3]

While Hispanics have made gains in education, according to the U.S. Census Bureau, they have recently faced setbacks in income levels. The census reported that Hispanic households experienced a real decline of 2.6 percent in median income between 2002 and 2003. The report states that a greater percentage of Hispanics, both nationals and immigrants, live in poverty, second only to African Americans (22.7 percent versus 21.4 percent) than before 2002.

Any discussion of obesity and poverty among minorities must take into account deeply embedded racism. Latinas, like African American women, come face to face with prejudice every day. For instance, a young Chicana may have to interpret English for her Spanish-speaking parents and consciously or subconsciously absorb a stranger's distain. Or, she may encounter people who hear her Spanish-flavored speech and automatically assume she's a domestic worker and/or not smart enough to speak English. (In the case of black Latinas, many people are dumbfounded that someone who looks African American can speak Spanish *and* English — twice as many languages as most white Americans speak.) Unfortunately, brown-skinned, Spanish-speaking people tend to be lumped together as either Mexicans or Puerto Ricans, without other distinct Latino cultures being acknowledged.

These prejudices are further reinforced by the media. The movies and evening news continue to promulgate negative stereotypes of Latinas, frequently depicting them reciting the rosary, whirling in a salsa dance, cleaning someone's house, using or dealing drugs, or barefoot and pregnant, madonnas or *la prostituta*.

Many Latinas aspire to alter public perceptions by becoming educated and qualified for jobs in which they can present more positive images. *Latina* magazine is an excellent example of a growing Hispanic media presence. Established in 1996, *Latina* has a circulation of over two hundred thousand. The bilingual publication explores lifestyle and fitness issues from a Hispanic American point of view.

Surgery across the Border

Many young, educated Latinas internalize the same body issues that black women do. Feeling pressure to conform to a model-thin body type, more and more Hispanic teens and women are developing eating disorders, such as bulimia, anorexia, and compulsive overeating. Also, increasing numbers of Latinas are seeking weight-loss surgery.

Like African Americans, Latinas often have less access than whites do to quality medical care to prevent and treat weight-related diseases. They're also more likely to experience mishaps and medical disasters.

The International Bariatric Registry reports that just three thousand Latinos had gastric bypass operations in 2003. However, as Latinas move into higher-paying jobs with medical insurance that will cover gastric bypass, the number of surgeries is sure to increase.

Meanwhile Dr. Alberto Aceves is the beneficiary of Latinas' interest in low-cost weight-loss surgery. He runs the Mexicali Bariatric Center in Mexicali, Mexico, where he has performed over 1200 "lap-band" procedures. His specialty is a minimally invasive surgical treatment in which he inserts a silicone band around the upper part of the stomach to create a new small pouch, a technique much like the Fobi pouch.

The cost of the procedure at the Mexicali center is just $8,200 — compared to $ 30,000 or more at hospitals in California. Dr. Aceves's weight-loss "package" includes "pre-op testing, services of the surgical team and anesthesiologist, a two-day hospital stay, transportation to and from the airport, and a two-night hotel stay for the patient and their companion."

Dr. Aceves warns potential patients, "If there is a complication, any extra medical charges are not included" in the basic price. He emphasizes that though "the risks of having problems [resulting from the procedure] are less than 2 percent [he claims to have had no complications]," for those willing to spend three days with him on the way to forever slender, "there is always a risk with any surgery."

Dr. Aceves's patients from the United States must sign consent forms that stipulate the same medical regulations and laws that govern U.S. surgeons do not bind hospitals or physicians like Dr. Aceves who practice outside of the United States. If something should go wrong, patients may have few if any legal remedies.

Carmen Makes a Life-Altering Decision

Carmen, the Orange County social worker, knew about Dr. Aceves, but decided to have her surgery closer to home. She had few doubts about her decision to have surgery though her husband of eighteen years, Roberto, was terrified at the prospect. After a few months, she convinced him that the alternative — remaining fat — was a sure death sentence. All her aunts and her mother died of diabetes caused by being overweight.

After researching the surgery for ten years, Carmen had the procedure in 2003, the same year her mother died. Her mother's death was the deciding factor.

Growing up in the Dominican Republic, she remembers her mother fixing huge meals for her family of three. "We always had enough to feed ten people for every meal. When my mother was growing up, a woman with round hips was considered beautiful. It was a completely different story when we came to America.

"It wasn't like my mother was poor growing up that caused her to have all the excess. She lived on a farm and there was always enough to eat. It has more to do with the Dominican culture. As a child I ate lots of vegetables and fruits on the farm, but we also ate lots of fried pork and beef. Everything was cooked with an abundance of oil and salt. But I was involved in baseball and volleyball and gymnastics."

When Carmen's family moved to the Bronx in 1976, everything changed. Her mom was afraid to let Carmen and her sister go outside to walk or play or enjoy the outdoors as they had in the Dominican Republic. The lack of exercise, combined with fatty, fried foods, wreaked havoc on her body. "I eventually got to be 340 pounds, and I am only five feet two," Carmen says.

She felt exhausted all the time and was terrified of developing diabetes like her mother and other women in the family. She tried lots of diets and none worked. "People say, 'Just go exercise,' but it's not easy to move around when you are so overweight," says Carmen. "I asked my personal physician if he would recommend me for the surgery and he said yes. He referred me to another doctor who luckily was part of my medical group so it all worked out and within a week my surgery was approved."

Convincing Roberto she should have surgery took time. "He kept telling me, 'Don't do it, I love you just the way you are.' But I told him I have two choices: One, I'll die on the operating table; or two, I'll die of diabetes because eventually I knew I was going to get that disease. I am glad I did something to prevent it."

Fortunately, Carmen did not have any problems with the surgery. However, she'll require additional surgeries to remove the loose skin, procedures she's not sure she can afford. She believes the best part about her operation is that it has completely changed her eating habits. "I don't eat red meat or sugar and I drink soy instead of cow's milk," says Carmen. "Now if I overeat — even one tablespoon — I feel it because I had the gastric bypass with the staples. So if I keep eating, it starts to hurt."

Hasta la Vista, Barbie

For the past two years, two thirty-something Mexican American psychologists have been holding up a mirror to hundreds of Los Angeles teens. By the end of the daylong session, young women begin to love what they see. Adios Barbie, a program designed by Dr. Denna Sanchez and Dr. Monica Rosas-Baines, helps young Latinas appreciate themselves and their bodies, focus on their positive achievements, and value education.

Adios Barbie takes its name from the 1998 collection of irreverent essays on body image, formerly entitled *Adiós, Barbie* (now retitled *Body Outlaws* after Barbie manufacturer, Mattel, raised objections). *Body Outlaws* features multicultural perspectives about the female body, distorted for over forty years, in the curvaceous doll with its anatomically impossible dimensions.

"In the U.S., we live in a consumer society where beauty can be bought in the form of expensive makeup, plastic surgery, costly diet plans, and gyms," says Dr. Rosas-Baines. "Many women from less developed Latin American countries don't have the luxury of worrying about their weight. There are greater concerns just to survive."

According to Dr. Rosas-Baines, young American women of color may feel that their skin color, hair type, body shape, and facial features are unattractive since they don't match the American female ideal. "It can lead a girl to feel bad about herself and ashamed of her ethnicity."

Both Dr. Rosas-Baines and Dr. Sanchez agree that signs of the unhealthy obsession many women have with their bodies and their weight are visible everywhere. "We see it with all women of all ages," says Dr. Sanchez. "Even when highly educated professionals gather, the conversation inevitably gets around to weight or dissecting body parts. This dialogue can begin as early as elementary school — when we start noticing boys, we start notic-ing other girls and comparing ourselves to them."

The Adios Barbie program was created to inspire women to challenge society's message of what's beautiful and to develop a positive self-image. In the sessions, the psychologists encourage young women to say goodbye to Barbie as a cultural icon of beauty and to welcome a personal view that includes self-acceptance and the acquisition of knowledge. With the psychologists acting as moderators, teens discuss the messages they receive from media, family, and friends about how they should look. Dr. Sanchez says, "One of the questions we ask is, 'How much time do we spend criticizing ourselves?' Whether they live in the inner city or in suburbia, all the students admit to being bombarded by a narrow image of what it means to be beautiful, and they spend lots of time feeling they have to measure up to this pre-imposed standard."

The psychologists discuss the detrimental effects of poor self-image, including feelings of shame, low self-esteem, insecurity, depression, eating disorders, and body dysmorphic disorder (a type of anxiety disorder that causes someone to become abnor-mally preoccupied with a real or imagined defect in her physical appearance). These all result from the fact that on some level the young women hate what they see when they look in the mirror.

The program includes a silent exercise to demonstrate atti-tudes toward body image. The girls are asked to stand on one side of the room or the other depending on whether they agree or disagree with certain statements:

- I am satisfied with my body shape.

- I have never dieted.
- I have been criticized by someone in my family about the way I look.
- When I look in the mirror, I do not like what I see.

"The exercise is extremely powerful," says Dr. Sanchez. "It helps the girls think about their own bodies and recognize that lots of other girls feel the same way they do. When we perform this exercise, most every girl moves to the 'agree' side for statements like 'I criticize myself about the way I look; when I look in the mirror I do not like what I see.' It's alarming to see how many girls feel so poorly about themselves."

Dr. Rosas-Baines adds, "There usually is a lot of uncomfortable giggling when the girls realize that so many of them are unhappy with their appearance." Afterward, the participants comment that they're surprised and saddened to see the number of girls who feel badly about themselves. They start to realize the effects negative thinking and outside influences have on their perceptions of themselves.

Developing a positive body image by becoming aware of negative self-talk and reorienting their focus to things that make them proud are the goals of Adios Barbie. Sanchez and Rosas-Baines recommend young women practice an optimistic mantra to encourage a positive body image. They encourage young women to stop competing with their friends for who has the fattest thighs, who has gained the most weight, who has the biggest behind, and so forth.

"We want women to feel empowered and take care of

themselves," says Dr. Sanchez. "We explain the 'garbage in/garbage out' theory of nutrition. We discuss the importance of taking care of your body by eating well and getting daily exercise."

At the beginning of each session, girls are given an index card to write the name of a female they admire and three qualities they admire in that woman. At the end of the seminar, participants are asked to share what they wrote. Most select women who've had a significant impact on their lives — mothers, other relatives, or teachers. They list qualities such as compassion, strength, intelligence, and courage.

"We talk about how the qualities of the people we care about are internal — in our hearts, our minds, our talents — not in the size of someone's waist," says Dr. Rosas-Baines.

Both psychologists believe young Latinas are positively influenced by the increase of Latinos in the media. *Real Women Have Curves*, a coming-of-age film featuring a young Chicana, is a recent hit. The story features a young woman who works in her family's garment factory and dreams of attending an Ivy League university.

"The movie is a good example of some of the pressures young girls face within their own families when they are overweight or want to break away from established family traditions," Dr. Sanchez says.

Dr. Rosas-Baines says, "We are seeing women like Jennifer Lopez, America Ferrera, Eva Longoria, and Salma Hayek, who are celebrated for their beauty. No longer do you have to be a thin, blue-eyed blond to be considered attractive."

As society is becoming more diverse, the definition of what is considered beautiful is expanding. Women like Jennifer Lopez and others embrace their curves and celebrate their culture. "It's a wonderful message to young women, particularly young Latinas," says Dr. Rosas-Baines.

Affirmative lessons from Adios Barbie are ones women of all shades and shapes can understand and appreciate.

Rob's Recommendations

*Body Outlaws: Young Women Write About Body Image &
Identity* (formerly entitled *Adiós Barbie*), edited by Ophira Edut, published by Seal Press, 1998, 2000, 2004.

Latina Realities: Essays on Healing, Migration, and Sexuality, by Oliva M. Espín, published by Westview, 1997.

Empowering Latinas: Breaking Boundaries, Freeing Lives, by Yasmin Davidds-Garrido, published by Penmarin Books, 2001.

Loose Woman, by Sandra Cisneros, published by Vintage Books, 1994.

Hollywood's Finest

Selena. Breakthrough role for Jennifer Lopez. 1997.

My Family, Mi Familia (1995); *Real Women Have Curves* (2002); and *Selena* (1997). All star versatile actress Lupe Ontiveros.

CHAPTER EIGHT

Before You Make the Call

Regain the Lost

Each ounce I gain increases pain, I have to choose
to want to lose, the best reward, I give myself
will not be from the fridge's shelf. But will be for
myself to see if I can lose what's eating me.

—E. JOYCE MOORE

WOMEN LIKE STEPHANIE, Camille, Virginia, and Debra believe, as Cathy once did, that they are skinny people trapped inside big bodies. Cutting away fat with weight-loss surgery will allow the sexier, more confident woman beneath the extra pounds to shine.

This inner being can cross her legs and turn a brother's head; she never scouts restaurant booths big enough to accommodate her. She doesn't scavenge scraps from her kids' dinner plates or gorge on junk food after the little ones have gone to bed. When she passes a mirror, she lifts her head, looks herself in the eye, and celebrates her reflection.

"We are just touching the tip of the iceberg when it comes

to understanding obesity," says Dr. Fobi, who has performed over eight thousand weight-loss surgeries, a quarter of them for black women. He believes obesity is "an epidemic," and insists it is important that we as a society "educate ourselves about prevention and focus on treatment for those who already are obese." Because of the prevalence of diabetes in overweight young children, Dr. Fobi urges parents and educators to examine our consumption of fast food, its easy access, and its impact on our health. He also stresses the importance of exercise for adults and children.

"Right now everyone has an opinion about obesity, but most of the so-called experts are wrong," he says. "We have to educate the doctors, the public health people, the schools, the politicians who make the policies, the young, the old, the intermediate. It's going to take a long time, but it's going to go faster than things have in the past because a lot of people are affected by obesity — the Internet and the global media help spread the word, which improves our knowledge of obesity."

Pound for Pound

Whether a woman has gained a few pounds with each birthday or has been fat her entire life, it's easy to see why the seemingly miraculous answer of gastric bypass surgery far outweighs any perceived risks. Having been fat since junior high school, Cathy chanted a mantra in the days leading up to her surgery, "Either I die on the operating table or I die from being overweight." I heard this reasoning over and over again from other women. Weight-loss surgery is not viewed as a get-thin-quick solution. It's a yearned-for way to win over the scales once and for all.

"There might be a lady who weighs 250 pounds and is happy with her weight," says Dr. Fobi. "She carries herself well, she functions, she exercises, and she stays fit. She is happily married. Weight-loss surgery is probably not a realistic or necessary option for her. Another person who weighs 190 pounds may be miserable with her weight. She's done everything to try and lose it, but she always gains it back. She's a better candidate because surgery will make her lose the weight and accomplish what she wants to in terms of slimming down. Trying to do surgery on somebody who is 250 pounds but sees no problem with it is doomed to fail because she's not going to comply with the requirements to keep the weight off."

The Triple Whammy

Being a female of color, a black woman already has two mighty strikes against her. Adding weight to the equation is strike three. Fat African American women often feel alienated from the mainstream, living life on the sidelines, gawked at or ignored. Sometimes they overcompensate by being "mama" to everyone, the "class clown," the "pissed-off sister" who throws her weight around, or a "nervous Nellie," needy and emotionally bruised. Whatever the role, they may binge on food, alcohol, recreational drugs, or sex (usually with the wrong men). Loved ones may insist, "You have such a pretty face, and what a great personality," or "You look fine the way you are," or "Black men love women with some meat on their bones." But fat black women know better: If those things are true, then why are skinny females getting all the good jobs and good men? They know that despite what people tell them, size discrimination is very real.

After all, overweight sisters rarely see anyone who looks like them on TV, on the silver screen, in music videos, or in fashion magazines. Heck, even talk show empress Oprah Winfrey is thin now. Many sisters confess they liked Oprah better when she was big and struggling with her weight—like them. It's no wonder some women will do anything to be thin.

"The complications from being overweight are physical, social, economic, psychological, and medical," explains Dr. Fobi. "For example, a woman who is extremely overweight is very likely to have aches and pains because of her size and overall health. Someone who is three hundred pounds may simply bend over and risk a back sprain or other injury."

Many of Dr. Fobi's patients are extremely high risk, severely obese people who must use breathing machines or walkers on a daily basis. And although it's illegal for employers to discriminate against a person because of a disability, Dr. Fobi says, "There will be economic consequences because they may be unable to find the job they're qualified to perform. In addition, the overweight or obese person will have a hard time getting medical or life insurance because companies classify her as a high risk."

Nonsurgical Remedies

Doctors, nutritionists, mental health professionals, and others who treat obese black women caution their patients against acts of desperation. Some medical experts believe reliance on gastric bypass surgery for weight loss is a dangerous trend and recommend nonsurgical steps that emphasize behavior modification and changing one's self-image. They see these solid, but less dramatic and invasive programs as more suited to achieving long-term health.

Dieting Roller Coaster

For cultural and physiological reasons, most diet trends don't work long term. Losing weight and keeping it off are daunting, but some weight-loss strategies tend to be more successful than others. For example, many doctors believe that black women should reject plans like the Atkins diet that emphasize low carbohydrates, high fat, and high protein. Many black women already suffer from heart disease, high blood pressure, and diabetes, conditions that can be exacerbated by this kind of eating. Other fad diets, expensive muscle-building exercise equipment, pills, powders, and drinks rarely result in long-term weight loss. Many women who tried so-called miracle concoctions, like the "forty-eight hour diet," and dropped up to ten pounds in a weekend's time can attest to the fact that they spent days feeling jittery and regained the lost pounds quickly.

Lasting weight loss comes with a change of mind and heart, improved eating habits, and regular exercise. This is true for women who seek surgical and nonsurgical programs.

"The only way to lose weight," says Dr. Kevin Brown, who treats obese black women in his Los Angeles general practice, "is to exercise more and eat less." Dr. Brown believes that in rare instances, gastric bypass surgery may be warranted, but is not a realistic option for most women. He has seen too many cases of distraught African American women who have regained weight after undergoing surgery.

The "eat less, exercise more" advice may seem like bunk to a sister who is one hundred pounds overweight, has tried every diet, never exercises, and wants a quick fix. But physicians like Dr. Brown are adamant that to achieve true weight loss, women must invest time in an overall health plan no matter what their current size. After all, says Dr. Brown, "if you can walk to the refrigerator, you can walk around the block." (A thirty-minute daily stroll is considered by experts to be the minimum amount of exercise for everyone, overweight or not.)

But suppose a woman is dying to see what it feels like to wear a tank top that slips easily over her breasts and a miniskirt that shows off her gorgeous legs, or wants to ride the roller coaster at Magic Mountain. Perhaps she has tried eating less and working out but doesn't stick with it long and gains even more weight. What then?

The Yellow Pages are full of insurance companies that may offer coverage for weight-loss surgery. Even so, cheaper, less drastic options for losing weight and achieving optimum health should be considered before going under the knife.

Weighing Your Options

There are a number of possibilities when it comes to weight loss. Before you choose, consider all your options:

Option 1: Discover whether you have an eating disorder.
Option 2: Turn to a power greater than yourself—the twelve steps of Overeaters Anonymous.
Option 3: See a psychologist or therapist who specializes in body image issues.
Option 4: See a nutritionist.
Option 5: Consider Weight Watchers, which for years has helped dieters watch portion size and exercise regularly.
Option 6: Look into medical fasting.
Option 7: Practice fat acceptance.

Option 1: Is Your Eating "Dis-ordered"?

Eating disorders usually conjure up visions of emaciated teens who stick their fingers down their throats and eventually wind up on television talk shows telling their stories. Few in the black community would associate an overweight sister, daughter, mother, wife, or friend who is always laughing and loves to grub with someone suffering from a medically recognized eating disease.

"Dis-ordered" eating behaviors like anorexia nervosa and bulimia have crept into the lives of young African American women and teens who are afraid of becoming obese. Conversely, experts estimate that around 5 percent of overweight or obese people suffer from a lesser-known eating malady called "binge eating disorder" (BED), also known as "compulsive overeating." Women with BED act like bulimics, who binge, get physically ill, and throw up. Afterward, bulimics dissolve into guilt and self-recrimination, and start the vicious cycle over again. Women with BED, like those who suffer from bulimia, consume huge amounts of food in a short period of time; unlike bulimics, BED sufferers typically do not purge. They, too, feel powerless to stop overeating, and experience a sense of shame following the binge. Like bulimics, compulsive overeaters consume food in secret, use food for coping with stress, and indulge when not hungry. Skeptics believe compulsive overeating is just an excuse for a woman who refuses to put down her fork. While the doubters may be right in some cases, for other women, BED is a genuine condition that can be treated.

Stephanie, the thirty-three-year-old student and single mom who used to refer to herself as "super-sized," realized she needed some kind of "intervention" to stop overeating. In 2002, she found a new medical insurance plan that covered gastric bypass. She had the operation, lost one hundred pounds, and is keeping the majority of it off. She believes she still has an eating disorder, though she was never officially diagnosed.

For example, before gastric bypass Stephanie constantly had what she calls "bad food" thoughts, referring to a concept of "good food" (fruits and vegetables) versus "bad food" (french fries and donuts) taught in many weight-loss programs. Stephanie would wake up in the morning obsessed with what she planned to eat that day. After wolfing down a four-course breakfast, she would snack until lunch, then nibble until dinner. Stephanie couldn't tell the difference between being physically hungry and just wanting to eat.

The day before surgery, Stephanie treated herself to one last secret binge, testing herself to see how many Big Macs she could consume. She ate four — but could have eaten many more. For Stephanie and other compulsive overeaters, food is rarely chewed or actually tasted and savored. After a bite or two, they just swallow.

Even today, after weight-loss surgery, Stephanie still has "bad food thoughts" and looks forward to pigging out at an all-you-can-eat Chinese buffet lunch with her naturally slender mother. Her "eyes are bigger than her stomach" at the buffet, and she gets full fast. But Stephanie says she can still consume many of her favorite foods, though not at one sitting like she once did. She is on guard, realizing that if she's not careful, she could easily gain back all her lost weight. Stephanie could probably benefit from eating-disorder counseling. However, since she's now at her goal weight, she feels she can control her eating — for now anyway.

Binge eating disorder can wreak havoc on a woman's physical and emotional well-being, leading to hypertension, diabetes, heart disease, a damaged gallbladder, and obesity. Women who engage in compulsive overeating experience tremendous guilt and shame, and sometimes have trouble forming lasting emotional bonds with others. Not all women who suffer from BED are overweight, and not all overweight women are afflicted with BED. A family doctor can make a referral to an eating-disorder specialist, and the Internet lists many as well. Among the professionals trained to treat BED are the following:

- Licensed marriage and family therapists (MFT)
- Licensed clinical social workers (LCSW)
- Medical doctors (MD)
- Registered dieticians (RD)

Recovery from BED can include individual, family, couples, and group counseling, inpatient and outpatient treatment settings, nutrition counseling, and medication. Insurance companies, HMOs, Medicare, and Medicaid sometimes pay for treatment.

There is also help for those struggling with BED at Eating Disorders Anonymous (EDA). Founded in 2000, EDA is a fellowship of men and women who meet to "share experience, strength and hope" and to recover from eating disorders like BED. Based on the principles of Alcoholics Anonymous, EDA provides support for people who want to recover from disordered eating in a confidential setting. It offers meetings in person and online. For more information, check out nationaleatingdisorders.org.

Option 2: Overeaters Anonymous—
One Day at a Time

Similar to EDA, Overeaters Anonymous (OA) uses the twelve steps and twelve traditions for recovery from Alcoholics Anonymous (AA). As described in Chapter Four, its goal is to help fat women and men develop a healthier relationship with food. Founded in Los Angeles in 1980, OA holds meetings daily across the country.

There are no dues or membership fees, and participants need not reveal their identities. No one checks to see whether you are following the program. OA members are encouraged to acquire a sponsor — another OA participant whom they can call on for support and a sympathetic ear. The OA message to people struggling with their weight is simply this: You do not have to go it alone.

Farlane, who was sexually abused by her childhood neighbors, is a true "friend of Bill W.," an AA-inspired reference to people involved in twelve-step programs. In trying to heal from her early trauma, Farlane joined AA, Cocaine Anonymous (CA), Narcotics Anonymous (NA), and Sex Anonymous (SA). Then she found OA, which she credits with helping her "get honest" about her dangerous behaviors, which included not just overeating, but engaging in unprotected sex and stealing from her employer. Farlane became deeply involved with the program, holding meetings in her home and traveling to different cities to share her experiences with other OA members. Over time, she lost one hundred pounds, and along with the weight, she shed many of the rationalizations for her self-destructive actions.

Like most anonymous twelve-step programs, OA maintains a philosophy of attracting members rather than promoting itself. To find out more about OA, go online to oa.org.

The Twelve Steps of Overeaters Anonymous

1. We admitted we were powerless over food — that our lives had become unmanageable.
2. Came to believe that a Power greater than ourselves could restore us to sanity.
3. Made a decision to turn our will and our lives over to the care of God *as we understood Him.*
4. Made a searching and fearless moral inventory of ourselves.
5. Admitted to God, to ourselves, and to another human being the exact nature of our wrongs.
6. Were entirely ready to have God remove all these defects of character.
7. Humbly asked Him to remove our shortcomings.
8. Made a list of all persons we had harmed and became willing to make amends to them all.
9. Made direct amends to such people wherever possible, except when to do so would injure them or others.
10. Continued to take personal inventory and when we were wrong, promptly admitted it.
11. Sought through prayer and meditation to improve our conscious contact with God *as we understood Him,* praying

only for knowledge of His will for us and the power to carry that out.

12. Having had a spiritual awakening as the result of these Steps, we tried to carry this message to compulsive overeaters and to practice these principles in all our affairs.

Option 3: See a Psychologist or Therapist Who Specializes in Body Image Issues

EDA and OA encourage sharing intimate thoughts and fears with the group on the road to recovery. This kind of public confession can be scary for black women because it contradicts lessons we learned growing up to avoid "airing dirty laundry" and to "keep our business to ourselves." Those old messages can make it difficult for us to open up to strangers about our pain and to discuss honestly how we feel about being fat.

There's also a fading stigma in the black community about seeking professional help for mental and emotional issues. No one wants to be called "crazy" by friends and family, if it's discovered that she is seeing a "head doctor." Besides, there's the stereotypical belief that all African American women have a better body image than other groups of women, even if they're overweight or obese. For some women this may be true, but it isn't the case for all, as evidenced by the increasing numbers seeking weight-loss surgery.

Also, many people mistakenly believe because African

American women have endured so much and are so emotionally strong, they're able to hold it together and are resourceful enough to simply "get over it" or figure a way out of any psychic hurt. It's stressful to deal with racism and economic injustice. And, as more and more black women become educated and affluent, they experience stresses that go along with high-octane lives and powerful paychecks. Psychotherapy and other forms of mental health counseling have become increasingly desirable for addressing overwhelming emotional issues like clinical depression. HMOs, health insurance plans, and community mental health centers make professional help available to many women. In addition, university or medical school programs often provide low-cost assistance, and local medical and/or psychiatric societies can help for little or no money. The Association of Black Psychologists has a website (abpsi.org) and helps connect African Americans to therapists who can place them on the road to well-being.

Option 4: See a Nutritionist

As Dr. Fobi explained in Chapter Two, genetics play a major role in obesity. It doesn't require genetic testing to know that lots of fat people in a family can indicate there's a genetic propensity for obesity. Even with the genetic component, however, a nutritionist can teach you how to eat in a healthier way, suggesting ways to combine foods, eat healthy snacks, and build awareness of the components of food that work best with your body and lifestyle. A nutritionist usually begins a consultation by running blood tests to assess cholesterol and sugar levels, testing for food and other allergies, and conducting a full or partial physical. She will work with you to prepare a daily "food diary" to chart your weight-loss progress.

Option 5: Weight Watchers

For the last forty years, one group in particular has become synonymous with dieting—Weight Watchers International (WW). A tried-and-true way to lose weight and maintain weight loss, Weight Watchers does not demand dieters give up favorite foods like pizza or fried chicken. Its program is based on a point system (all foods are given numerical values) and encourages eating in moderation and never starving. WW also suggests walking for regular exercise.

Similar to EDA and OA, WW holds meetings daily at which weight-loss "winners" share their triumphs with other WW members. Guest speakers are usually people who have lost fifty pounds or more (and maintained the weight loss).

Unlike the anonymous fellowships, WW isn't based on twelve guiding principles and sponsorship is not required. However, weigh-ins occur at every meeting, and members can privately measure weight-loss achievements or share their goals with the group if they so choose.

Hearing the slow and steady progress of the WW success stories inspires black women like Lee, a twenty-four-year-old teacher's assistant who tried Jenny Craig, liquid diets, and sporadic "fasting." Still trying to lose fifty pounds, Lee first attended WW when she was a teenager but could not relate to the "sob stories" of people much older than she was at the time. These days Lee understands that folks attend the meetings because they "love to eat and that is mostly the reason we are overweight."

Lee likes the fact that at twelve dollars a week, with no special foods to buy, Weight Watchers fits into her part-time-job budget. She says the difference between WW and other programs is that WW relies exclusively on formerly overweight people who have remained thin to convey realistically how a person loses weight and keeps it off. For example, before she returned to WW, Lee used to polish off a twenty-piece box of McDonald's Chicken McNuggets a couple of times a week. Following WW recommendations, Lee says she still enjoys McNuggets, but now she gets a six-piece box once a week and breaks them in half to extend the eating experience.

Best of all, WW is nonjudgmental; if you happen to gain a couple of pounds over a week or don't exercise for a couple of days, "No one is there to put you down or make you feel weak," says Lee.

WW meetings are held in most communities. WW also has a "corporate solutions" plan that companies can offer their employees. For more info, log on to weightwatchers.com.

Option 6: Is Medical Fasting What the Doctor Ordered?

Who could forget Oprah pulling her red wagon full of fat? In the late 1980s, the talk show queen waged a very public battle with her weight and rolled a cart of lard on stage to represent all the pounds she had lost on a liquid diet. Oprah's weight loss that time was short-lived, but millions of dieters took heart in her ability to fast her way to a size 8.

Some experts view such an extreme diet (properly known as a protein-supplemented modified fast) in the same dim light they do weight-loss surgery. Sometimes called a "starvation diet," patients under a doctor's supervision are forbidden from eating any food for at least thirty days. Instead patients subsist on a protein drink that includes vitamins and minerals. After a period of time, ranging from two to fourteen weeks, the patient is gradually guided back to solid foods, all the while being counseled on how to eat a healthier diet and exercise regularly. It's not unusual for patients to lose up to fifteen pounds in a week though much of the initial weight loss is in fluid loss. After the first week, weight loss is usually kept at below 1.5 percent of body weight per week.

The obvious drawback of this kind of weight-loss plan is its restriction against eating anything for the first few weeks. Most people find it impossible to do, even with close medical supervision. Dr. Michael Myers of weight.com in Los Alamitos, California, opposes the widespread use of weight-loss surgery as a first option for weight management. Instead, he offers various treatment options for his patients ranging from working with a dietician and exercise physiologist to utilizing a "protein-sparing modified fast liquid diet plan." Having worked with obese patients since 1980, he believes that although much of the weight loss occurring with a gastric bypass can be maintained over a long period of time, most physicians and patients are unaware of the long-term nutritional deficiencies that develop and the need for continued monitoring and treatment to avoid both short-term and long-term complications.

Dr. Myers believes obesity is like other chronic illnesses that can be controlled but not cured. He thinks the best that patients can hope to lose and maintain on any medical reducing program is around 20 to 25 percent of their total body for severely over-weight individuals; for less severe forms of obesity, total weight loss is usually closer to 10 percent.

The ideal candidate for medical fasting is someone with a BMI of 30 or above, who has other obesity-related health conditions such as hypertension and diabetes, and has unsuccessfully tried other traditional diet approaches.

Oddly enough, a new relationship has developed in recent years between gastric bypass surgery practitioners and proponents of medical fasting. Because many people are advised to lose weight *before* having surgery, companies like OPTIFAST, a manufacturer of liquid diets, now tout the benefits of their products with the claim that if a patient can get used to a "highly restrictive" diet before surgery, it will be easier for them to adjust to eating less afterward. In addition, OPTIFAST purports to assist in the healing process "to preserve lean body mass during weight-loss surgery and improve immunity."

Because of the cooperative relationship between doctors who prescribe liquid diets and gastric bypass surgeons, it would be wise to ask if your doctor is in such a *quid pro quo* arrangement, and how the combined program may affect your overall health — and finances.

Medical fasting is expensive. HMOs like Kaiser Permanente offer a liquid-diet plan for about $100 a week for seventeen weeks, and private practitioners like Dr. Myers accept medical insurance. For more information on liquid diets, contact weight.com.

Option 7: Just the Way You Are—Fat Acceptance

Founded in 1969, the National Association to Advance Fat Acceptance (NAAFA) fights discrimination against fat people and provides "the tools for self-empowerment through public education, advocacy, and member support," according to its mission statement. Working to increase awareness about the "sociological, psychological, legal, medical and physiological facts of being fat," NAAFA charges nominal fees to join and holds local meetings and activities, such as advocacy workshops and activist support groups.

Vehemently against all forms of weight-loss surgery and dieting, NAAFA urges fat people to cease spending time and money trying to be thin. Through its literature, meetings, public relations, and advocacy programs, NAAFA advances the "radical" notion that fat people should accept and cherish themselves just the way they are and enjoy life to the fullest, supported by loving friends and family. Not all of us were meant to be the same size, the group believes. The important thing is that we strive to maintain the best possible health, regardless of what the scales and society say.

NAAFA believes the increase in obesity and eating disorders of late is the result of dieting. According to Debra Perkins, vice president of NAAFA's Los Angeles chapter, dieting causes the body to set up a defense system that forces it into a starvation mode making it burn "fuel" or food more efficiently. This reaction causes the metabolism to slow down. Regardless of whether the stomach and intestines are cut and reconfigured via gastric bypass, the metabolism essentially remains the same. In addition, NAAFA maintains that extended dieting thrusts the body into "survival mode," which produces cravings and causes unrestrained eating and overeating. The reason people gain weight when they stop dieting, says NAAFA, is because the body's mechanisms develop "insurance" against further starvation by adding on extra pounds. Most people rarely lose 25 percent of their diet goal before they reach a "plateau," and this stalling in the weight-loss process can happen with or without gastric bypass surgery.

NAAFA recommends that when choosing a weight-loss program, people look into two important issues: a documented five-year follow-up study that substantiates weight-loss claims and a money-back guarantee. Few dieters maintain their weight reduction beyond five years and NAAFA says the "consult your doctor first" disclaimers to dieters are really just a way to legally protect the multibillion-dollar diet industry against lawsuits when their diets fail.

Dr. Fobi and NAAFA represent polar opposites when it comes to opinions about the desirability of gastric bypass as a means of weight loss. But they agree on one thing: the failure rate of most diets. According to Dr. Fobi, studies reveal that diets fail 99 percent of the time. "And in five years, they will fail 110 percent of the time, because not only do people gain all the lost weight back, they usually gain more than 10 percent in addition," Dr. Fobi says.

In the opinion of diet experts like Dr. Myers, yo-yo dieting does more harm than good. Each time you gain and lose weight, you lose not just fat but water and lean muscle tissue too. When you regain, you gain back mostly fat. Therefore, as you lose and regain, you actually put your health at greater risk than by maintaining a higher weight and not dieting.

NAAFA also recommends that people seek the help of nutritionists and dieticians for maintaining a healthy weight, believing that they are better equipped to assist with weight-loss plans and strategies than are medical doctors. NAAFA takes the position that overweight does not automatically equate to poor health. They point to the fact that many thin people suffer from cancer, heart disease, and diabetes. And should you find yourself dealing with weight-related diseases, NAAFA recommends controlling them through medications, because dieting may worsen the illness. In addition, the anxiety, stress, and frustration resulting from failed diets do nothing to improve your mental or emotional health.

The NAAFA dictum is to accept yourself at your current size, stay active, and get on with your life. International Size Acceptance Association (ISAA) and Council on Size and Weight Discrimination (CSWD) have an activist focus similar to that of NAAFA. If you're ready to give up the battle of the bulge and get involved, log on to naafa.org.

Rob's Recommendations

Something's Wrong with Your Scale! by Van Whitfield, published by Anchor (paperback), 2000. A romantic novel about African American characters struggling to accept their weight.

Zami: A New Spelling of My Name, by Audre Lorde, published by Crossing Press, 1983. A coming-of-age story set in New York City with a protagonist who is lesbian, black, and overweight.

Big Girls Don't Cry, by Donna Hill, Brenda Jackson, Monica Jackson, and Francis Ray; published by Signet, 2005. Sexy stories with big, bold, beautiful women.

Hollywood's Finest

Super Size Me. Morgan Spurlock's scathing, Oscar-nominated documentary on the evils of the fast food industry and its marketing campaigns targeting children. 2004.

CHAPTER NINE

Generation XXXL

*There can be no keener revelation of a society's soul
than the way in which it treats its children.*
—NELSON MANDELA

GROWING UP IN the 1960s, before high-fat, salty, sugar-laden fast foods forever altered the appetites of Americans, Cathy was considered "pleasingly plump." By today's standards, she was far from obese or even overweight. Nor did she possess the outward confidence exhibited by many heavyweight teens of this generation. Maybe her lack of self-esteem caused us to tease her about her size. Or maybe our teasing diminished her confidence. Whatever the cause and effect, teasing was part of our dynamic. My siblings and I would taunt her with "Fatty Cathy" and "fat pig." Cathy never forgot. Nor did I. However, she remembered it more as a physical assault than a verbal one, and used to introduce me to her friends by saying, "This is my sister Robyn; she used to beat me up when we were kids."

Nowadays America's double message is everywhere. On one hand, young women are encouraged to be big, bold, and proud of who they are (and spend lots of money on clothes and junk food). On the other hand, society's message is unwavering: You can never be too rich or too thin.

Just as Cathy once idolized Marilyn Monroe, Shenay identifies with and adores famous shapely women. A witty eleven-year-old, she lip-syncs in front of the mirror, pretending to be Janet Jackson. She dances and dreams to the sounds of the sexy singer with the big breasts, tiny waist, and perfect life. In Shenay's make-believe world the screams of thousands of fans ringing in her head don't belong to Janet, they belong to her.

The only child of a slender telephone company manager, Shenay also satiates herself by eating her favorite foods like Cheetos Flamin' Hot and double-stuffed Oreos. She says her mother yells at her to stop eating, even berating her in front of family members. Pointing to Shenay's belly, her mother agonizes that her "little girl" is too young to have so many stretch marks and will end up with diabetes.

Shenay ignores her mother, along with the bathroom scale, which never moves past the 200-pound mark anyway. The biggest kid in her sixth-grade class, she is called "Fatty," "Shamu," and "baby Huey" by some of her classmates. Cookies and chips ease the pain of teasing but not the aches in Shenay's lower back and knees, pains she has a hard time talking about. Food and pretending to be Janet Jackson are the two things that make her feel good no matter what. Desperate and embarrassed, Shenay's mother has quietly been researching weight-loss surgery for her daughter.

An Obsession Is Born

April, an African American freshman in psychology at the University of Minnesota, attended her first Weight Watchers (WW) meeting when she was thirteen years old. At four feet eleven and 185 pounds, she — like many children — didn't realize she was overweight. Now eighteen, April doesn't recall being taunted on the playground or at home with her three brothers because of her weight. But she recalls her aunt and mother, both of whom are overweight, plying her with cautionary tales of how tough high school is for a "fat girl." They would "warn me that I would not be able to date or wear cute clothes," she remembers. "It all went in one ear and out the other."

April went to her first Weight Watchers meetings as a way to hang out with her mother and get away from her brothers. There she began to see weight as an issue in her life; she lost weight and has kept it off.

"I cry and get depressed if I gain one pound," April admits. Even though her high school senior class validated her talent and beauty by voting her prom queen, April's mom shakes her head, knowing the torment and angst April goes through because she "still thinks like a fat person."

Fat Camp

Nora, an African American stay-at-home mother of six, got the scare of her life when she took her daughter Tanya, then thirteen, for her annual physical. The doctor told her that Tanya had "borderline" high blood pressure. Frantic, Nora and her sister (who also has an overweight teen) scoured the Internet and found Camp LaJolla, a "fat camp" designed for children that was featured on *The Oprah Winfrey Show*. Tanya spent a summer vacation there and lost twenty pounds in five weeks.

After Tanya came home, she lost another twenty pounds, having adopted a new eating and exercise regimen. Now, she is the family "food cop," according to Nora, helping to prepare healthy foods for her siblings by "eye-balling" portions and making sure they eat as many vegetables as they want and avoid Hot Pockets, Popsicles, and frozen pizzas. Nora reports she too has lost twenty pounds, inspired by her daughter's new attitude toward food.

A Mother's Prayer

In her early fifties, Renee says she doesn't have much longer to live. She's not as troubled about her impending death as she is worried sick about what will happen to her twelve-year-old daughter, Yolanda. Renee has cried and prayed and begged and hollered for someone, some agency, some miracle to help her help her daughter lose weight.

Renee suffers from various ailments that have doctors baffled and keep her weak, her weight now down to eighty-five pounds. As Renee grows smaller, Yolanda gets bigger. In Renee's words, her daughter "has enough rolls of fat to fold her entire hand over. . . . Her stomach is like a road map of stretch marks even though she's not even fourteen."

Despite the tragedy befalling her mother, Yolanda seems unfazed. "She walks around like she owns the world," Renee laments. Watching Yolanda you would never guess she's already undergone heart surgery and has health problems beyond the worst fears of most parents.

"I'm terrified," says Renee. "Even though Yolanda has a baby face, older men flirt with her because she's so physically developed, with big breasts and wide hips. The fellas think my baby is grown. What's going to happen to my child when I die?"

Shock Waves

These are just a few of the faces of childhood obesity that threaten the future health of the African American family. From the halls of Congress to local school districts to suburban and inner city homes, we are a nation experiencing collective shock at the increasing numbers of overweight and obese children. Adults are rushing headlong into damage control to stem this epidemic that threatens the lives of millions of young people. Research reveals that there are more African American children with diabetes, heart disease, and obesity than ever before. But this crisis didn't land on our doorstep overnight. Children's weights have been trending upward for at least a decade. Some experts have even gone so far as to predict that unless the obesity rate among all children is reduced, the current generation (so-called "Generation XXXL") may be the first ever in U.S. history whose life expectancy will be *shorter* than that of their parents.[1]

African American and Latino children have been particularly hard hit by the childhood obesity crisis. According to the American Obesity Association fact sheet "Obesity in Youth," almost 36 percent of black children between the ages of six and eleven are overweight, and more than 19 percent are considered obese. Among twelve- to nineteen-year-olds, 40 percent are overweight and nearly 24 percent are obese.

Mexican American children fare even worse. Nearly 40 percent of Mexican American children ages six to eleven are overweight and almost 24 percent are obese.

Talk the Talk, Walk the Walk

While the problem of overweight and obese kids is overwhelming and getting worse, parents can play a vital role in helping them achieve and maintain a healthy weight. Some proactive tips include the following:

- *Know all you can about weight-loss surgery before you take that most extreme step.* Weight-loss surgery performed on kids was once considered taboo. But quiet as it's kept, more and more fearful parents are resorting to surgery as a means of achieving quick weight loss for their children. If the procedure is dicey for adults, it's a double risk for teens and preteens. Most bariatric surgeons won't operate on anyone under the age of eighteen. However, there are doctors who will perform weight-loss surgery on children as young as eleven years old. The most common procedure used for young patients is the lap-band method, approved by the FDA in 2001. (See Chapter Six for more on this procedure.) A minimally invasive technique, lap-band surgery is completed in about an hour and requires an overnight stay in the hospital. According to the National Institutes of Health (NIH), this procedure should only be considered for adolescents who are severely overweight:

Surgical treatment [should] only be considered when adolescents have tried for at least 6 months to lose weight and have not been successful. Candidates should be severely overweight (BMI of 40 or more), have reached their adult height (usually 13 or older for girls, 15 or older for boys), and have serious weight-related health problems such as type 2 diabetes or heart disease. . . .[2]

The NIH strongly recommends that both parents and patients be evaluated to see how emotionally prepared they are for the operation and for the lifestyle changes necessitated by the procedure. Because the procedure is relatively new, long-term effects on young minds and bodies are not yet known.

- *Form a support group for parents and guardians of overweight kids.* Having a forum for sharing and venting can help ease the emotional strain of raising an overweight child. To find interested members, post a notice at PTA meetings, at church, or at work. Set a weekly meeting time in rotating homes, if possible (no children allowed of course), and encourage participants to share anecdotes and insight about their struggles. While these meetings are for adults, let your children know what you are doing. Kids appreciate knowing that you consider their health a priority, and they may be more likely to go along with changes in family eating and exercise routines that you propose. Children's obliviousness about their weight is a common frustration for parents raising fat kids. Nagging, pleading, making deals, and breaking promises are traps many parents fall into. A support group can help parents find solutions that may make the difference between raising a healthy child and raising one who acquires a life-threatening disease because of her weight. It's also healthy for adults who are in the same boat to listen and empathize.

- *Teach your children by setting a good example.* The "Do as I say not as I do" school of parenting contributes to the problem of obesity. If you want your child to develop healthier eating habits and to value exercise, model that behavior. Consider making small changes in your routine that your child will notice: Pack a healthy homemade lunch rather than eating out at work, make and keep doctors' appointments, or park the car farther away from the store and walk.

To help our children with weight problems requires retraining ourselves — dropping old eating habits and sedentary lifestyle choices. You'll find that kids can adapt to change a lot easier than we set-in-our-ways adults. This is a good time to let children know that you're struggling to make changes to achieve better heath and that being overweight is not a moral failing.

- *Make healthier lifestyles a family affair.* Nora, the mother of six who sent her daughter to camp, recalls how the whole family drove eight hours from Northern California to San Diego to take Tanya to Camp LaJolla. When they arrived, Nora noted that of the two hundred kids in Tanya's age group about forty were African American. She saw children of all races as young as seven years old who were attending the program because they were already overweight or obese. When Tanya returned home from camp, the entire family underwent a lifestyle shift.

Nora cooks differently now, not using butter but a butter substitute, eliminating salt, substituting mustard for mayonnaise on sandwiches. "When we have french fries, we don't fry them," Nora says. "We put them in the oven. I used to cook vegetables and drown them in butter. Now I cook vegetables with just a little bit of water to get them warm. We eat a lot more vegetables and a lot more salads. I try new vegetables like asparagus and zucchini. I've cut out all gravy and sauces — no more smothered chicken. We bake or grill all of our meats."

Tanya makes all of the plates, controlling portions. She's become so adept at "eye-balling" that she can tell whether a piece of meat is four ounces, the healthy size. Ketchup is the family's best friend now. Says Nora, "We like it, but because it's high in sugars we limit how much of it we eat. Every now and then I will cook one of our old favorites like lasagna. It's okay to eat lasagna and tacos sometimes. Tanya has taught our family it's not really what you eat, but how much you eat."

- *Integrate physical activity into your family's daily routine.* Climb stairs instead of taking the elevator, walk your child to and from school when possible, find a family bowling league, or include a game of volleyball or basketball in your weekend barbecues. Go bike riding, swim, or jump rope. These are all activities that even some of the young members of the family can participate in and benefit from.

Many black families cite finances as a reason their children are overweight and lead a sedentary life. Gyms and exercise equipment are not cheap. And it is more expensive to eat healthy foods, for example fish. Sending a child to camp is well beyond the means of many families. Nora, however, was committed to getting Tanya the help she needed and says the entire family took part in efforts to raise the $6,000 it cost to send Tanya to Camp LaJolla.

"We sold raffle tickets, had bake sales, and we even had

a garage sale to make money for Camp LaJolla," Nora says. The lessons about food and exercise Tanya learned have benefitted the whole family.

"We have what I would call the 'fat gene' in my family," says Nora. "Most of the women in my family are overweight, so being fat was something we took for granted. But both my sister and I have overweight daughters and we knew we had to do something radical to stop the cycle."

Unfortunately, Nora's sister was unable to raise the last $2,000 to pay for the camp. "Money is definitely a big issue," says Nora. "But I thought about it this way: I would pay anything to help Tanya if she got heart disease or some other life-threatening illness. How much would I pay to keep from having to visit my child in the cemetery?"

Camp empowered Tanya and the whole family. Before that, Nora's mother-in-law and aunt often talked to Nora about Tanya's weight. "I would tell them, 'I hear you. . . . I know she's fat, but I don't know how to help her.' It was really frustrating because everyone would criticize, but they wouldn't offer solutions. Then one day I realized how fat she was and I thought to myself, 'Wow, something has got to give here.'" Nora tried to change her cooking and she took her daughter to Overeaters Anonymous.

But nothing was as successful as Tanya's experience at Camp LaJolla. "It was a jump start," Nora says. "Now we have the tools we need and the motivation to keep going. If I had to advise other parents, I would tell them not to force their children to diet, but to be supportive and encouraging of their struggle. If they aren't losing weight as quickly as you want, be patient, because eventually with the right program the weight will come off."

- *Praise even the smallest changes in behavior your child makes on her path to healthier eating.* The whole family must reevaluate how they relate to food. For example, suggest your child eat a baked potato instead of french fries. Even a child as young as six or seven years old will understand if you explain to them that "fried foods are bad for them." If your kids are older, let them know you notice their efforts to eat healthier and to exercise daily. Remind them that what they choose to eat today will affect the way they live tomorrow and beyond.

Tanya and her family decided to do something about her weight problem when she was still in middle school. Now at fifteen, Tanya is a candidate for a "camp counselor in training"; she will help newcomers on their journey to becoming slim teens. When Tanya turns eighteen, she will be eligible to be a regular camp counselor.

"At Camp LaJolla we exercised and we learned how to portion our food," says Tanya. "They taught us about nutrition and why it's so important to be healthy. I have lost a total of forty pounds. I want to keep dropping weight. It's not easy: My school doesn't serve the best food in the cafeteria — pizza and chicken nuggets, stuff like that.

"I knew I was overweight because my doctor told me. Plus, I was having pain in my joints, my knees and my ankles," Tanya continues. "Since I've lost weight, my joints don't hurt anymore and I exercise every day. Sometimes I use exercise videos at home, and I swim and play basketball at school.

"If I could talk to girls my age, I would tell them to lose weight for themselves, not for anyone else. Once you start losing weight, you feel encouraged to keep on losing. I would tell them not to give up . . . when you lose weight, people tell you, 'Wow, you look really good, you look really great.' But you have to change your eating habits. Now when I go to McDonald's I know I need to get a small fry instead of a king-size. Now I get a half cheeseburger instead of a whole one. Losing weight really brings up your self-esteem. Plus you get to buy lots of new clothes."

- *Educate yourself and your child about how the human body functions and teach her how to read food labels.* Make a family lesson plan to learn about serving sizes, fat grams, cholesterol, sodium, carbohydrates, and proteins, and how these food components impact one's emotional and physical well-being. Learn why it's important to drink eight glasses of water a day, exercise at least thirty minutes seven days a week, and eat fruits and veggies instead of candy and salty chips for snacking. *Dr. Gavin's Health Guide for African Americans,* by Dr. James Gavin, is a great reader-friendly handbook to help you start a dialogue with your kids about their health. *Patti LaBelle's Lite Cuisine: Over 100 Dishes With To-Die-For Taste Made With To-Live-For Recipes,* co-written by the world-famous singer Patti LaBelle, offers fun and delicious meals the family can create together.

Listen to your kids when they share how they feel emotionally. Is their overeating tied to being stressed, anxious, worried, or scared? Point out the connection between negative feelings and overeating. Suggest your children do something else if they are feeling frustrated or mad, like exercising.

- *Let your children know about diseases, such as hypertension, cancer, and diabetes, that run in the family.* The object here is to enlighten and inform, not to scare. Speaking openly and honestly will help kids be better educated about choices they make for their own lives. Let them know why not all foods are for everybody, and that food allergies are a real problem for African American kids. You don't have to be a doctor to discuss in simple language how the liver and kidneys function and why it's so important to maintain a healthy heart. With this knowledge and your encouragement and example, they will understand why it makes sense to snack on an apple rather than a Snickers bar.

- *Start a vegetable garden.* Planting food crops like tomatoes and onions can be a project for the whole family. You can plant seeds in your backyard or in planters along the windowsills. Give youngsters the opportunity to feel the earth between their fingers and watch plants sprout and grow from seedlings into healthy food. Children will learn lessons about nature they can use in the classroom to understand the nutrients in the foods they eat.

Don'ts and Dos

When frustration builds and all the nagging doesn't work, parents often turn to words and deeds that only make matters worse. Consider this list of don'ts before you do or say something you'll regret in the morning:

- *Don't tease or berate your child for being fat.* Some parents believe that by calling attention to their child's weight in an angry, disapproving way, the child will have an incentive to lose weight. Not only will this strategy fail, it can be tremendously damaging. A child does not become overweight in a vacuum; adults around her play a role in accepting, teaching, or passively allowing poor eating, nutrition, and exercise habits. If you nag, sooner or later your daughter will either tune you out or secretly eat more to ease the sting of your criticism. Let her know she is loved and beautiful. If she is obese, share in words and deeds the attitude that the problem can be solved. All family members should offer a young person who struggles with her weight support and love on the journey to better health.

- *Don't use food as a reward or a punishment.* What aggravated parent has not bribed a fussy child with candy as an incentive to calm down? It's as natural as holding her small hand when crossing the street. We adults have been taught to treat food as an indulgence: "To live to eat rather than eat to live." One L.A. couple considers it a "treat" to take their five kids to McDonald's every week for "Fish Friday," fillet-of-fish sandwiches fried and smothered in tartar sauce on sale for a buck a piece. They see this as killing two birds with one stone — feeding the family on the cheap and rewarding the children with an evening out. Unhealthy food offered as an incentive for good behavior can backfire. Children can be just as thrilled with a family outing that consists of a healthy meal and a chance to bowl or play miniature golf. If parents demonstrate they value the idea of family togetherness as much as they do going to McDonald's for empty-calorie foods, children will respond.

Our children's physical well-being depends on us making healthy choices. The goal is not to bombard children with scary information. Make the topics of healthy eating and exercise part of your daily dialogue. Kids will grow up to be well-informed adults and choose their meals wisely.

Weight and nutrition issues give us a unique opportunity for a black history lesson, exploring the relationship between African Americans and food, why we store much of what we eat today (whereas in the past we burned it, through more physical activity), and why an overabundance of fast food is harmful to everyone's health.

- *Do not chain or lock the refrigerator.* Why turn your child into a food bandit? One overwrought black mom was so frustrated with her inability to get her overweight five-year-old to stop eating, she padlocked her refrigerator when the child was old enough to open it on her own. At one point, the youngster threw a tantrum, trying to unlock the food. Meanwhile the mother wears the key around her neck as though she's a jailer.

Not only is a locked refrigerator in the family kitchen unsightly, hiding food reinforces the idea in a child's mind that food is "bad," that they're being punished, or that something very valuable exists behind the door, making the kid want it even more.

Discussing healthy eating habits and practicing what you preach are better solutions. Refrigerators with nutritious, good-tasting snacks — low-fat, low-sugar yogurts, apples, tangerines, carrots, celery, low-fat peanut butter — reinforce healthy eating and make it unnecessary to hold food as a prisoner in your home. If you don't want your kids to eat junk food, don't buy it.

- *Avoid buying or cooking so much food that you wind up throwing away leftovers.* One homeless sista swears that she eats better than most from the well-stocked trash cans around Los Angeles. We take the availability of food for granted. But in most of the world, food and water are precious commodities. Part of teaching our kids healthy habits involves showing them how to be responsible citizens of the world and make sensible choices about many things, including food.

Americans throw away hundreds of tons of food every day. While that isn't a crime, it reflects poor values and money management. Some African Americans who grew up poor feel compelled as successful adults to have big spreads at every meal. As understandable as that is, it doesn't make up for the pain of having been a hungry child. Nor does it teach our children healthier habits. Remember the old admonition to eat everything on our plates because "children are starving in Africa"? Millions of children around the globe still go to bed hungry every night. Consider the message we send our kids when we cavalierly throw food away. It's time we heed another one of grandma's favorite sayings: Waste not, want not. One sister bags her leftovers and leaves them outside on top of the trash. She says they're always gone before the end of the day.

In an era when so many African American children are overweight, it's time we change the way we cook — not only what and how we prepare food, but the amount we cook and consume every day. Experts say the first step on the road to better eating is to eat smaller portions. Teaching our kids that bigger is not always better is a great way to lessen or ward off childhood obesity.

When You Know Better, You Do Better

Children become overweight or obese for the same reasons adults do — eating too much and exercising too little. In his book, Dr. Gavin points out some of the warning signs and reasons that a child might be developing a weight problem: abnormal weight gain as a toddler, consuming too much fried food, drinking too many sugary soft drinks, skipping meals, heredity, and not enough exercise. Here are some strategies to address each problem:

- *Abnormal weight gain between the ages of three and five.* Talk to your pediatrician about low-sugar, low-sodium foods, and never use candy to quiet a fussy child.
- *Consuming too many fried and starchy foods.* Replace sweets and starches with fresh fruits and vegetables, lean meats (like chicken and fish), nuts, and grains. Serve smaller portions.
- *Drinking too many sugary soft drinks.* Drink six to eight glasses of water a day, and limit the amount of sugary juice and soda in the house.
- *Skipping meals.* Make sure your child eats three balanced meals daily. Consider this rule of thumb for adults: "Eat like a king for breakfast, eat like a queen for lunch, and eat like a pauper for dinner." Because children burn more fuel, they get hungry during the day. Let them tell you when they're hungry, rather than the other way around. Get rid of the Gummy Bears and beef jerky, and provide nourishing snacks like carrots, celery, and cucumbers instead.
- *Sedentary lifestyle.* Encourage children to exercise at least thirty minutes every day. Hula hoop, basketball, tetherball, kickball, jogging, hopscotch, and jumping rope are old-school activities that burn calories and are fun, even for the video-game generation.
- *Heredity.* If hypertension, diabetes, and other weight-related diseases run in your family, be sure your child has regular checkups to monitor her heart, weight, blood sugar, cholesterol levels, and overall health.

The Dangers of Kid Fat

Know the life-threatening health risks for children carrying too much weight or reaching obesity in youth:

- *Type 2 diabetes.* This condition used to be called adult-onset diabetes, before health-care professionals started seeing large numbers of children in middle school who had acquired or were on the verge of developing this life-threatening condition. African Americans, Hispanics, Native Americans, Asian Americans, and Pacific Islanders are at greater risk for this kind of diabetes, according to the American Diabetes Association. The disease is particularly worrisome in children because it can lead to kidney failure, nerve and eye damage, and heart disease. There is no cure for diabetes in children or adults but it can be controlled with a change of lifestyle, diet, exercise, and medication. The most common symptoms of diabetes in children are
    * Frequent urination
    * Excessive thirst
    * Extreme hunger
    * Unusual weight loss
    * Increased fatigue
    * Irritability
    * Blurry vision

    If your child is complaining of any of these conditions, seek medical help immediately.
- *Asthma.* The number of African American children with asthma

has quadrupled in the last twenty years due to a combination of increased air pollution, old homes with environmental problems, and poor eating habits.

- *Hypertension.* According to the American Obesity Association, persistently elevated blood pressure levels occur nine times more frequently in obese children and adolescents (ages five to eighteen) than in children of normal weight.
- *Sleep Apnea.* A condition in which a person stops breathing during sleep, sleep apnea occurs in about 7 percent of children with obesity. The combination of obesity and sleep apnea in children can lead to neurological problems, according to the American Obesity Association.
- *Long-term psychological and social effects.* Being an overweight child can take a devastating toll on one's mental health. It all begins with teasing. No matter how much you try to protect her, your child must go out into a world where other kids as well as many adults feel it's okay to verbally assault someone because of her size.

  According to many psychologists, verbal harassment in childhood often leads to severe depression, post-traumatic stress disorder, anxiety, and social phobias (or social anxiety disorder). Negative coping patterns such as drug and alcohol abuse are often the consequences of childhood teasing. Children mocked for being fat, for example, sometimes display a measure of self-hatred by making fun of themselves. This helps them mitigate the hurt and lack of self-confidence they may feel.

Teasing is often the result of historical racism in African American culture, according to Dr. Tiffany Herbert, a university psychologist who uses group therapy as a means of empowering young black women. It recalls an era when African Americans were pitted against one another; taunting became a way to show superiority and assert one's individuality. "We as African Americans have historically been taught that European culture is the standard of beauty, wealth, socialization, and other traits perceived to be so-called 'right,'" Dr. Herbert says. Taunting someone for being fat or for some other perceived flaw often reflects the low self-esteem of the bully and may be a manifestation of internalized racism. "The idea is to make someone feel as bad as you feel on the inside," says Dr. Herbert. "And through taunting, the teaser gains some level of superiority over someone else."

Being the target of name-calling often has a profound impact on a person's sense of self, her gender, or her race. It can also create a beneath-the-surface rage that may eventually explode violently.

It Takes a Village and a New Nutrition Vision

Tracie Thomas, assistant director of Student Nutrition Services at the Compton Unified Schools, sees firsthand the damaging effects poor eating habits and lack of exercise have on black and Latino children. She has discovered that one way low-income children can receive better nutrition is for educators and farmers to join hands. In addition to working daily to educate children, teachers, and parents about the importance of good nutrition and regular exercise, Thomas is changing the eating habits of young people. She has put salad bars filled with fresh fruits and vegetables in every elementary, middle, and high school in the Compton district. Featured in the *Los Angeles Times* and on *CBS Evening News*, she has a long-range vision for every school in America to have a salad bar in its cafeteria. Then children can choose nutritious eating at the very place where they spend much of their young lives.

Thomas believes the obesity crisis in the black community will not be solved by just eating fewer Big Macs. She advocates setting up long-term programs focusing on nutritional counseling and physical education, programs that will help this generation escape the fate of many of their parents.

"I think the most serious complications are the chronic illnesses that occur at such an early age," Thomas says. "In addition, black children aren't receiving the education and knowledge of healthy eating habits at school. As a result, many aren't engaged in physical activity.

"When I talk to parents, I ask them, 'How many of you used to walk to school?' Just about every hand goes up. It's a lot different now . . . parents are afraid to let their children walk even a few blocks to school."

Thomas continues, "There is even a lack of awareness among teachers of how harmful the lack of exercise and the consumption of high-fat, high-sugar foods are for children. I tell parents and faculty that this generation is literally killing themselves with their forks."

Faced with grim and mounting statistics of childhood obesity in the African American community, Thomas puts her passion and vision for healthy kids in motion with a plan she urges school districts across the country to adopt.

Her salad bar program, set up in 2004, serves produce from California farms. Thomas and other advocates of "Farm to School" programs (including the U.S. government) believe this is a win-win situation: "Children have the opportunity to eat fresh, healthful lunches, and small and medium-size farms are guaranteed the schools' business," says Thomas.

Thomas suggests the following steps for parents and school officials interested in offering a salad bar program or other nutrition-education programs in their region:

- Encourage teachers to integrate healthy foods in subjects they already teach, like math, history, and social science. For example, one Compton middle-school math instructor keeps apples and other fruits on hand to explain fractions. She then gives the fruit to her students as a snack.
- Set up regular meetings at school with parents to discuss the importance of good nutrition for the entire family.
- Contact a local farmer or food cooperative directly or a food broker who can act as liaison between farmers and the school districts.
- Ask health-care organizations to donate pedometers that

allow students to keep track of the number of steps they take each day.

- Research how to use commodity foods, surplus produce, cheese, meat, and other items from the USDA to ensure the salad bar meets federal nutritional requirements for school lunches. Those resources can help keep the cost down.

- Investigate federal and state grants that can help pay for healthy food programs like the salad bars.

"Good nutrition is a balance of consuming healthy foods and physical activity as a lifestyle," Thomas says. "It's okay to eat other less healthy choices like fast food, but only in moderation."

The family that doesn't know better believes they are getting a better deal by feeding five kids for $5.95 at McDonald's than by purchasing food and fixing a balanced meal on a daily basis. "Unfortunately," says Thomas, "that's the best some low-income families can do."

While Thomas agrees that obesity begins with the kinds of foods black people are raised eating, she believes that with the amount of education available today about the importance of good nutrition and exercise, there's no excuse for children to be so overweight.

She dismisses the "show me a fat child, and I will show you an overweight adult" axiom. While obesity can be hereditary, it doesn't have to be. Some studies show that a parent's obesity is the greatest risk factor for obesity in children, but this doesn't mean that genetics are the sole factor responsible. According to a 2004 study at Johns Hopkins, "sixty-four percent of 9.5-year-old children with overweight parents became overweight compared with 16 percent of those with normal-weight parents. The authors hypothesize this connection is due to a combination of genetics and family environmental influences. . . ."[3]

Many fat children have parents who are not overweight, however. "I don't believe overweight adults produce overweight children," Thomas says, citing the example of her own family — her husband is a vegan and yet her ten-year-old daughter struggles with her weight. "The reason black children are overweight goes back to the lack of physical activity, too much consumption of fast food, fewer whole-food meals being cooked at home, eating too much processed meat, and super-sizing everything.

"Add to that the elimination of physical education programs in middle and high schools around the country and the current generation's fascination with electronic couch-potato gadgetry, and that sets the stage for a lifetime of health problems."

Starving to Be Thin?

A dangerous and potentially deadly way some African American girls deal with their fear of becoming obese is by using extreme dieting to stay slim. Some college and high school girls literally starve themselves.

As has already been discussed, research on body image among girls has found that African Americans tend to be more satisfied with their bodies than are Caucasians. Perhaps because of the positive, self-accepting attitude many young black women display, scant attention has been paid to African Americans who suffer from eating disorders. One exception is the *Ricki Lake Show*, which in 2003 devoted an entire hour to the problem of anorexia and bulimia among African American teens.

Many of the young women I advise readily admit to using diet pills daily, experimenting with colon cleansers, using laxatives, skipping meals. They routinely experience fainting spells, exhaustion, and irritability because of going full days without eating.

Christine, a carmel-skinned former college homecoming queen, recalls that when she was a high school freshman she teetered on the brink of an undiagnosed eating disorder. "I would drink a cup of coffee with my grandma in the morning and then go to school," Christine remembers. "At lunch when everyone else was eating, I would 'borrow' a french fry and eat it." She isn't sure whether she was medically anorexic since "black folks don't like to go to the doctor." Now overweight, she traces her food problem to when she began "restricting" certain foods like sweets and later stopped eating altogether.

"My mother saw I had a problem," Christine recalls. "So she started literally spoon-feeding me whatever our family was having for dinner. She had to force food on me because I just wouldn't eat. It got to the point where I could not eat because my stomach would hurt when I did."

During her sophomore year of high school, she started to eat again because she'd given up trying to lose weight. "I went from eating nothing to eating everything."

Now in her early twenties, Christine says she is "concerned" but not overly worried about her weight. "High blood pressure and diabetes run in my family," she says, "so no matter what I weigh, I figure I'm going to get one of those diseases regardless."

April, the coed from Minnesota who cries every time she gains a pound, also has a love/hate relationship with food. A size 7, she has gained seven pounds since starting college and is "really worried about it. . . . The hardest part for me is I can't stop eating. Even when I'm full, I won't stop eating. I eat and eat and eat. If I'm not hungry, I eat. If I'm bored, I eat. If I don't want to do something, I eat. I just discovered this pattern and I am trying not to do that so much."

April doesn't throw up after these binges, though one of her aunts is getting suspicious because April "picks at her food and immediately goes to the bathroom." Christine, on the other hand, admits to "vomiting" and taking diet pills during her high school years.

Neither April nor Christine has a healthy relationship with food. Both girls treat food as an enemy with the power to destroy them. As young black women go to college and move into the professional world, the pressure to be perfect and mold themselves into images similar to their white counterparts is tremendous. Is it any wonder some African Americans take their weight battle to another level?

Parents who think their children may be suffering from anorexia, bulimia, or any other eating disorder should watch for the signs described in Chapter Four and seek medical attention right away.

Our children's future depends on the choices we adults make. Living in a world where excesses and conveniences can make us sick, we yearn with a child's impatience for a quick cure when our bodies expand or begin to break down. As we transform ourselves from the inside out, our bodies, minds, and spirits will reflect a new and lasting peace.

Rob's Recommendations

Patti LaBelle's Lite Cuisine: Over 100 Dishes With To-Die-For Taste Made With To-Live-For Recipes, by Patti LaBelle and Laura Randolph Lancaster, published by Gotham, 2004.

Smart Parenting for African Americans: Helping Your Kids Thrive in a Difficult World, by Jeffrey Gardere, published by Dafina Books, 2002.

The Black Parenting Book, by Allison Abner, Linda Villarosa, and Anne C. Beal, published by Broadway Books, 1998.

Raising Black Children, by James Comer and Alvin Poussaint, published by Plume, 1992.

Hollywood's Finest

Fat Albert. Features a positive, upbeat representation of a big African American kid and his buddies, both animated and real-world. 2004.

Shrek (2001)and *Shrek II* (2004). The greatest fairy tales "never told" deliver the message of love and self-acceptance to kids of all ages.

Afterword

After the Hunger

A SUDDEN DEATH in a family changes everything.

When Cathy died, our family collapsed. Four years later we are still rebuilding our emotional lives.

A few months after Cathy died, Luke began dating again. In 2005, Luke married a woman from El Salvador. As the surviving spouse, he received the six-figure settlement from the doctors responsible for Cathy's death. Soon after receiving the check, Luke sold the home he, Cathy, and their children shared for a fraction of what it was worth — eager to move on and start a new life. Most of Cathy's enormous collection of antiques, clothes, family pictures, mementos, furniture, and the entire Marilyn collection was given away, thrown away, or sold. Luke and his new wife are raising Cathy's adopted daughter, and have no contact with me or other members of our family.

On the bright side, both of Cathy's stepdaughters have had babies, Cathy's grandchildren. For Cathy's parents, sisters, brother, nieces, nephews, aunties, uncles, and cousins, life goes on, the memories of her laugh never far from our minds. A group of Cathy's closest friends still meets on her birthday and the anniversary of her death. They usually go to one of her favorite restaurants then to her gravesite in Riverside to say their hellos. They always invite me to go, but I can't.

Cathy's death was foretold the first time she looked in the mirror and decided she didn't like what she saw. Many of the women I spoke to while writing this book reminded me so much of my sister. Through them I gained a better understanding of Cathy, her inner pain, and why she made the choices she did.

During the course of writing this book, Linda B. — who was determined to have a gastric bypass — changed her mind. Instead, she lost weight by cutting back on her favorite foods and taking up line dancing. "It's safer to lose weight this way," Linda B. says. "Plus, I am having fun."

I am sure if Cathy knew her own story helped someone like Linda B. move closer to self-acceptance, she would have embraced Linda B., shed a few tears, and invited her to her next party.

Cathy lived with optimism, joy, hope, and a special love for children. So, when you think of Cathy, please smile. She was a really cool sister.

See you 'round the way.

Notes

INTRODUCTION

1. "If a group calling itself the 'Center for Consumer Freedom' were to take out $600,000 worth of newspaper advertising claiming that the link between smoking and mortality is nothing but 'hype,' it would be a national scandal or, perhaps, just a national joke. . . ." *Washington Post* Editorial. Page A16. May 2, 2005.

2. "Diet and physical inactivity accounted for 400,000 deaths in 2000, or about 16.6 percent of total deaths. Tobacco, with 435,000 deaths, was 18.1 percent of the total, says research in today's *Journal of the American Medical Association*." "Obesity on Track as No. 1 Killer" by Nanci Hellmich. *USA Today*. March 4, 2004.

3. "Disputed Obesity Study Slipped Through CDC Filters: Inquiry shows scientists had objected to the report, which may have exaggerated death rates," by Rosie Mestel. *Los Angeles Times*. February 10, 2005. Page A20.

CHAPTER ONE

1. "Gastric Bypass Surgery Gone Bad," www.cbsnews.com/stories /2005/01/21/earlyshow/contributors/melindamurphy/main668323 .shtml.

2. "Roux-en-Y gastric bypass for morbid obesity — Home Study Program," Association of periOperative Registered Nurses (AORN), *AORN Journal*, by Cynthia J. Barrow. Page 593. 2002.

3. "However, white women experienced BD (body image) discrepancy at a lower BMI level (BMI = 24.6), and below the criterion for over-weight (BMI = 25). In contrast, black and Hispanic women did not

report BD until they were overweight (BMIs of 29.2 and 28.5, respectively)." "The Relationship Between Body Image Discrepancy and Body Mass Index Across Ethnic Groups," by Marian Fitzgibbon, Lisa Blackman, and Mary Avellone, North American Association for the Study of Obesity. 2000.

4. "More U.S. Schools Cut Gym," *Detroit Daily News.* October 15, 2003.

CHAPTER TWO

1. *Fast Food Nation: The Dark Side of the All-American Meal,* by Eric Schlosser, Perennial. 2002.

2. *The Obesity Myth: Why America's Obsession With Weight Is Hazardous to Your Health,* by Paul Campos, Gotham. 2004. Chapter Five: "The King's Two Bodies." Page 89.

3. *The Fat Girl's Guide to Life,* by Wendy Shanker, Bloomsbury. 2004. Page 193.

4. "Obesity in Minority Populations," American Obesity Association, AOA Fact Sheets. 2002.

5. *Las Sergas de Esplandián* (The Exploits of Esplandian), by Garci Ordóñez de Montalvo, first published in Seville, Spain, in 1510.

CHAPTER THREE

1. "Marital Status and Health United States 1999–2002," by Charlotte Schoenborn, MPH, Division of Health Interview Statistics. Abstract published in "Advance Data from Vital Health Statistics," Centers for Disease Control, Number 351. December 9, 2004.

2. "African American Men's Perceptions of Body Figure Attractiveness: An Acculturation Study," by Tammy Webb, Joan Looby, and Regina Fults-McMurtery. "This study examined African American men's perceptions of body figure attractiveness based on their acculturation levels. . . . Results revealed . . . that African American men perceived women with smaller body figures as more attractive than women with larger body figures." *Journal of Black Studies.* Vol. 34, No. 3, pages 370–385. January 2004.

3. *Stolen Women: Reclaiming Our Sexuality, Taking Back Our Lives,* by Dr. Gail Wyatt, Wiley. 1998. Chapter Two, page 33.

NOTES

CHAPTER FOUR

1. *Black Rage*, by William H. Grier and Price M. Cobbs, Bantam Books 1968. Page 67.
2. *No Secrets, No Lies: How Black Families Can Heal from Sexual Abuse*, by Robin Stone, Harlem Moon. 2004. Page 39.
3. "The Effects of Childhood Sexual Abuse on the Adult Survivor," Survivors of Incest Anonymous. 1998.
4. "What You Can Expect from OA," Overeaters Anonymous. 1998–2004.

CHAPTER FIVE

1. "The Cultural Image of the African American Woman," published in the *Birmingham-Pittsburgh Traveler*. http://northbysouth.kenyon.edu/2000/women/mammypage.htm.
2. *Stolen Women: Reclaiming Our Sexuality, Taking Back Our Lives*, by Dr. Gail Wyatt, Wiley. 1998. Chapter Two, pages 31–32, 33.
3. Ibid.
4. "Black Viewership Mystery Deepens," by John Consoli. "Black women viewers are popping up in the oddest of places across the TV landscape, and sometimes missing from the very places they historically have been found, namely UPN. . . ." *Mediaweek*. December 13, 2004.
5. *Skinny Women Are Evil: Notes of a Big Girl in a Small-Minded World*, by Mo'Nique and Sherri A. McGee, Atria 2003. Page 1.

CHAPTER SIX

1. "AIDS Conspiracy Beliefs Strong Among U.S. Blacks." Laura Bogart, a behavioral scientist for the RAND Corporation research group and a coauthor of the study. Interviewed on National Public Radio's "News & Notes with Ed Gordon." January 27, 2005.
2. "Study: Racial Health Gap Persists." "A recent study by former Surgeon General David Satcher says health in communities of color has improved considerably over the last fifty years. But, there still exists a chasm between black and white mortality rates. According to the report, more than 83,000 African-Americans die each year as a result of pervasive inequalities in America's social, economic and health-care systems." National Public Radio's "News & Notes with Ed Gordon." March 17, 2005.

199

3. "Substantial racial and ethnic disparities exist in health insurance coverage. In 2002, some 10.7 percent of working white, non-Hispanic Americans were uninsured, compared to 20.2 percent of working African-Americans, 18.4 percent of working Asians, and 32.4 percent of working Latinos. The risk of being uninsured is particularly high for immigrants who are not citizens: 43.3 percent of non-citizens were uninsured." Center on Budget and Policy Priorities, "Number of Americans Without Health Insurance Rose in 2002." October 8, 2003.

4. "Key Questions to Ask Before Having Bypass," by Tracy Correa. *Fresno Bee*. September 23, 2002.

5. Letters to the Editor. *Fresno Bee*. January 23, 2003.

6. "Key Questions," by Tracy Correa. *Fresno Bee*.

7. www.nhlbi.nih.gov/guidelines/obesity/e_txtbk/appndx/appndx8.htm

CHAPTER SEVEN

1. "Beyond Burgers: While McDonald's stomps on rivals around the world, its U.S. business has plateaued. Can pizzas and teriyaki burgers save the day?" by Bruce Upbin. *Forbes* magazine. November 1, 1999.

2. "Study Links Obesity to U.S. Residency: Study Finds Obesity Rare in Foreign-Born Until They Have Lived in U.S. for More Than 10 Years": "Long-term exposure to American culture may be hazardous to immigrants' health. A new study found that obesity is relatively rare in the foreign-born until they have lived in the United States — the land of drive-thrus, remote controls, and double cheeseburgers — for more than 10 years. . . . 'Part of the American dream and sort of life of leisure is that you also have some of the negative effects, and obesity is one of the major side effects of the success of technology and just having a life of leisure,' said [study's] co-author Dr. Christina Wee of Harvard Medical School. 'It's a double-edged sword.'" Abcnews.com. December 15, 2004.

3. www.obesity.org/subs/fastfacts/obesity_minority_Pop.shtml.

CHAPTER NINE

1. Jay Olshansky, a researcher on weight and aging: "We think today's younger generation will have shorter and less healthy lives than their parents for the first time in modern history unless we intervene." Reported on cnn.com. March 20, 2005.

2. "Gastrointestinal Surgery for Severe Obesity," *National Institutes of Health Publication for Health Care Professionals*; Weight-control Information Network. 2005.

3. "Predictors of Body Fat Gain in Non-Obese Girls with a Familial Predisposition to Obesity." By M. S. Treuth, N. F. Butte, J. D. Sorkin. *American Journal of Clinical Nutrition*. December 2003. 78(6): 1212.

Where to Get Help

Alcoholics Anonymous (AA)
P.O. Box 459
Grand Central Station
New York, NY 10163
(212) 870-3400
www.alcoholics-anonymous.org

American Cancer Society
(800) ACS-2345 (800-227-2345)
www.cancer.org

American Diabetes Association
1701 N. Beauregard Street
Alexandria, VA 22311
(800) DIABETES (800-342-2383)
www.diabetes.org

American Heart Association
7272 Greenville Avenue
Dallas, TX 75231
(800) AHA-USA-1 (800-242-8721)
www.americanheart.org

**American Society for
Bariatric Surgery**
100 S.W. 75th Street, Suite 201
Gainesville, FL 32607
(352) 331-4900
www.asbs.org

**American Society of
Hypertension**
148 Madison Avenue, Fifth Floor
New York, NY 10016
(212) 696-9099
www.ash-us.org

American Stroke Association
7272 Greenville Avenue
Dallas, TX 75231
(888) 4-STROKE (800-478-7653)
www.strokeassociation.org

**Association of Black
Psychologists**
P.O. Box 55999
Washington, DC 20040-5999
(202) 722-0808
www.abpsi.org

Black AIDS Institute
1833 W. 8th Street, Suite 200
Los Angeles, CA 90057
(213) 353-3610
www.blackaids.org

**California Black Women's
Health Project**
101 N. LaBrea, Suite 610
Inglewood, CA 90301
(310) 412-1828
www.cabwhp.org

Center for Media Literacy
3101 Ocean Park Boulevard,
Suite 200
Santa Monica, CA 90405
(310) 581-0260
www.medialit.org

**Centers for Disease Control and
Prevention**
1600 Clifton Road
Atlanta, GA 30333
(404) 639-3311 or (800) 311-3435
www.cdc.gov/netinfo

**Council on Size & Weight
Discrimination**
P.O. Box 305
Mount Marion, NY 12456
(845) 679-1209
www.cswd.org

Curves International
100 Ritchie Road
Waco, TX 76712
(800) 848-1096
www.curvesinternational.com

Ebony Overeaters Anonymous
ebonyoa.home.att.net

Mal Fobi, MD
Center for Surgical Treatment of
Obesity
(800) 564-3624
www.cstobesity.com

**International and American
Associations of Clinical
Nutritionists (IAACN)**
15280 Addison Road, Suite 130
Addison, Texas 75001
(972) 407-9089
www.iaacn.org

**International Size Acceptance
Association (ISAA)**
P.O. Box 82126
Austin, TX 78758
(512) 371-4307
www.size-acceptance.org

Kaiser Family Foundation
2400 Sand Hill Road
Menlo Park, CA 94025
(650) 854-9400
www.kff.org

Magic Johnson Foundation
9100 Wilshire Boulevard
East Tower, Suite 700
Beverly Hills, CA 90212
(310) 246-4400 or (888) MAGIC-05
www.magicjohnson.org

Michael D. Myers, MD
Obesity Specialist
10861 Cherry Street, Suite 300
Los Alamitos, CA 90720
(562) 493-2266
www.weight.com

**National Association for the
Advancement of
Colored People (NAACP)**
4805 Mount Hope Drive
Baltimore, MD 21215
(877) NAACP-98 (877-622-2798)
NAACP 24-hour hotline: (410)
521-4939
www.naacp.com

**National Association to Advance
Fat Acceptance (NAAFA)**
P.O. Box 188620
Sacramento, CA 95818
(916) 558-6880
www.naafa.org

**National Coalition of 100 Black
Women**
38 W. 32nd Street, Suite 1610
New York, NY 10001-3816
(212) 947-2196
www.ncbw.org

**National Eating Disorders
Association**
603 Stewart Street, Suite 803
Seattle, WA 98101
(206) 382-3587
www.nationaleatingdisorders.org

National Institutes of Health
9000 Rockville Pike
Bethesda, MD 20892
(301) 496-4000
www.nih.gov/health/infoline

**National Latina Health
Organization**
3507 International Boulevard
Oakland, CA 94601
(510)534-1362
www.latinahealth.org

**National Mental Health
Association**
2001 N. Beauregard Street, 12th
Floor
Alexandria, VA 22311
(703) 684-7722 or (800) 969-
NMHA
www.nmha.org

ObesityHelp
(866) WLS-INFO
www.obesityhelp.com
Founded in 1998, this is the
Internet's meeting place for information and resources on obesity
and weight-loss surgery.

**Obesity Law and Advocacy
Center**
1392 E. Palomar Street, Suite
403-233
Chula Vista, CA 91913
(619) 656-5251
www.obesitylaw.com

Office of Minority Health Resource Center
P.O. Box 37337
Washington, DC 20013-7337
(800) 444-6472
www.omhrc.gov

OPTIFAST
(800) 662-2540
www.optifast.com

Overeaters Anonymous
(505) 891-2664
www.oa.org

Spelman College Women's Research & Resource Center
350 Spelman Lane, Box 115
Cosby Hall, 2nd Floor
Atlanta, GA 30314
(404) 270-5625
www.spellman.edu

Survivors of Incest Anonymous
World Service Office
P.O. Box 190
Benson, MD 21018-9998
(410) 893-3322

Taking Off Pounds Sensibly (TOPS)
www.tops.org

WebMD Health
669 River Drive, Center 2
Elmwood Park, NJ 07407
(201) 703-3400
www.webmd.com

WeightWatchers.com
(800) 221-2112
www.weightwatchers.com

YWCA USA
1015 18th Street, Suite 1100
Washington, DC 20036
(202) 467-0801
www.ywca.com

Group Topics and Discussion Questions

1. In just two years, the number of black cosmetic-surgery patients has grown by almost one-third, according to the American Society of Plastic Surgeons, jumping from 375,025 in 2002 to 487,887 in 2004. How does changing your physical features relate to your sense of black pride? If someone has a nose job, does that make her any less black?

2. Discuss the statement: "Black men like big women." In your experience, is this true? Who seems to perpetuate this statement? What role does the media play in determining beauty and what is considered sexy? What is the "tyranny of ideal"? How do you feel about interracial dating?

3. Which women do you look up to most? Why? If they include celebrities, what qualities do you admire most? Discuss the images of black women on television, in videos, and in movies. What do they have in common? How much diversity do you find?

4. What gives you "the blues"? Do you use food or alcohol to cope when you are feeling bad? Who do you talk to when

you feel overwhelmed? Discuss the statement: "Black women are sensitive."

5. Is your hair a source of racial pride? Have you ever worn your hair naturally? Does your hair interfere with your ability or desire to exercise regularly? What were the positive and/or negative messages you received in and outside of your family about your hair?

6. Discuss the statements below. Afterward, talk about the ways that your self image determines how you talk about yourself and behave toward others.
   a. I am satisfied with my body shape
   b. I have never dieted
   c. I have been criticized by someone in my family about the way I look
   d. When I look in the mirror I do not like what I see.

7. Discuss your eating habits. Do you eat when you are bored, lonely, happy, feeling celebratory, or needing a reward? How hard would it be change what and when you eat?

8. How do you feel about fast food restaurants in poor inner-city neighborhoods? How do the advantages outweigh the disadvantages in terms of African American health? In terms of employment opportunities?

9. What can be done about our overweight kids? Discuss ways black children can become fitter and develop better eating habits.

10. In what ways are African American women and Latinas similar? Discuss your views on black women from other places, such as Africa or the Caribbean. Do you feel a natural bond or a sense of unfamiliarity? What ways can woman come together across racial and cultural lines?

11. The griot or storyteller is an important conduit of information in African and African American culture. Discuss why it is important for black people to "tell our own stories."

12. Would you choose gastric bypass surgery to lose weight? Why or why not?

Acknowledgments

MY GOD.

To my daughter, Natice, for her laugh-out-loud honesty and for helping me to reveal and honor Auntie Cathy. Tee, it was you who kept my head out of the clouds and my fingers on the keyboard. Thanks for being so patient with Mom and "that book." I love you madly.

My parents William and Orelda; siblings Claudia, William, Jr., Sheilah, and Theresa; the next generation Geoffrey, Salena, Beth, Katie, Rodger, Patrick, Alex, December, Brett, Eric, Lil Chris, Micah, Beka. Uncle Stan, Auntie Betty, Eva, and Esther. William Wilks, Sr.

The Richardson family, especially Leya, Grandma Mona, and Leona, the Sacramento McGees, with a special shout out to my writing cuz, Marc, and Mo Mo's memory, Anita.

Anne, Bridgett, Loni, Nichole B, and Angie W, Jackie B, Jennifer and Pat Holley, I wanna thank you. To the crew from the Women's Center for their love and encouragement: Amanda, Lee, Lynn, Keena, Delcia, Kendra, Gladys, Riem, Shanice, Xica,

Michelle, Natasha, Haleemon, Angela, Theo, James, Connie, Morris, Anita R, and Victoria M. My students at the California Design College; and my online truth-seekers at Black Writers United.

California State University, Dominguez Hills' finest: Dr. Hansonia Caldwell, Dr. Joyce Johnson, Dr. Patricia Cherin, Dr. Thomas Giannotti, Dr. Howard Holter, Dr. Margaret Blue, Dr. Susan Fellows, Dr. Larry Ferrario, Dr. Iset Anuakan and Dr. Timothy Chin, Dr. Monica Rosas-Baines, Dr. Denna Sanchez, Dr. Tiffany Herbert.

For Alice: love and appreciation for sharing memories of Missy, who, like Cathy, took a risk and died too young.

Brooke Warner and Jill Rothenberg for recognizing and honoring my vision. Thanks to my agent, Jacky Sach, for her doggedness and patience.

Cathy's best friends Patty and Verdawn; attorney Michael A. Lotta, Bobby Samuels, Judy from Jazzy and Farah, Sherri from B&N, and Master Harris.

Friends of Bill W known and unknown.

Sonia Sanchez and Elizabeth Nunez — thanks for opening my eyes to this story.

The North Country Institute and Retreat: Dr. Tony M, Kari, Stephanie, Ohene and Rodney, Alex, Dr. Brenda Greene, Dr. Wesley Brown, Dr. Indria Ganeson, and thanks to Marie for sharing so much savvy.

Marie and Grover Deary of "2000 Plus"; California African American Women's Health.

All the women I interviewed for this book who fearlessly opened their hearts and shared their lives with me, especially Farlane, Sandra C, Jackie, and Stephanie. You were truly Cathy's voice.

Pat, Stan Jr., Uncles Benny and Richard, and Rachel. RH, what can I say? Thanks for everything. In loving memory.

Index

About the Author

ROBYN McGEE is currently the Director of Women's Resources at California State University, Dominguez Hills. McGee frequently writes and lectures on women's issues and popular culture.

McGee has a bachelor's degree in journalism, a minor in black studies, and a master's degree in humanities with a literature concentration from California State University, Dominguez Hills. In 2004, McGee received the coveted "Woman of Distinction" award. She has had articles published in *Seventeen* magazine, the *Black World Today*, Hearst Publications, and *Fireweed* feminist journal.

McGee and her daughter live in Southern California. You can visit her on the web at www.robynwrites.com.

Selected Titles from Seal Press

For more than twenty-five years, Seal Press has published groundbreaking books. By women. For women. Visit our website at www.sealpress.com.

The Black Women's Health Book: Speaking for Ourselves edited by Evelyn C. White. $16.95, 1-878067-40-0. Featuring Alice Walker, bell hooks, Toni Morrison, Byllye Y. Avery, Audre Lorde, Faye Wattleton, Jewelle L. Gomez, Marian Wright Edelman, and many others, this pioneering anthology addresses the health issues facing today's black woman.

I Wanna Be Sedated: 30 Writers on Parenting Teenagers edited by Faith Conlon and Gail Hudson. $15.95, 1-58005-127-8. With hilarious and heartfelt essays from writers such as Dave Barry and Barbara Kingsolver, this anthology will reassure any parents of a teenager that they are not alone.

I Will Survive: The African-American Guide to Healing from Sexual Assault and Abuse by Lori S. Robinson. $15.95, 1-58005-080-8. This valuable resource for survivors — and their families, friends, and communities — walks readers through the processes of emotional, physical, sexual, and spiritual healing, and the particular difficulties African Americans face on their journey toward recovery.

Waking Up American: Coming of Age Biculturally edited by Angela Jane Fountas. $15.95, 1-58005-136-7. Twenty-two original essays by first-generation women — Filipino, German, Mexican, Iranian, and Nicaraguan, among others — describe the complexities of being caught between two worlds.

Autobiography of a Blue-Eyed Devil: My Life and Times in a Racist, Imperialist Society by Inga Muscio. $15.95, 1-58005-119-7. The newest manifesta from the best-selling author of *Cunt* this time tackles race in America.

Nervous Conditions by Tsitsi Dangaremba. $15.95, 1-58005-134-0. With irony and skill, this novel explores the devastating human loss involved in the colonization of one culture by another.